SAS Clinical Programming

In 18 Easy Steps

FOR M.Pharm / M.Sc (Life Sciences) /M.sc (Stats)/ M.C.A/M.Tech / B.Pharm /Bio-Tech/B.Tech.

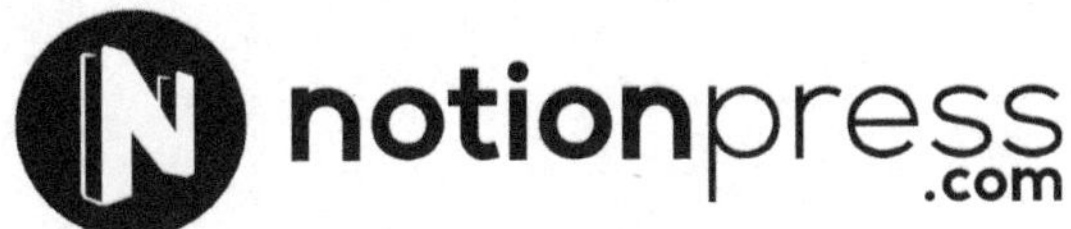

SAS Clinical Programming

In 18 Easy Steps

FOR M.Pharm / M.Sc (Life Sciences) /M.sc (Stats)/
M.C.A/M.Tech / B.Pharm /Bio-Tech/B.Tech.

Mr. Y. Lakshmi Prasad

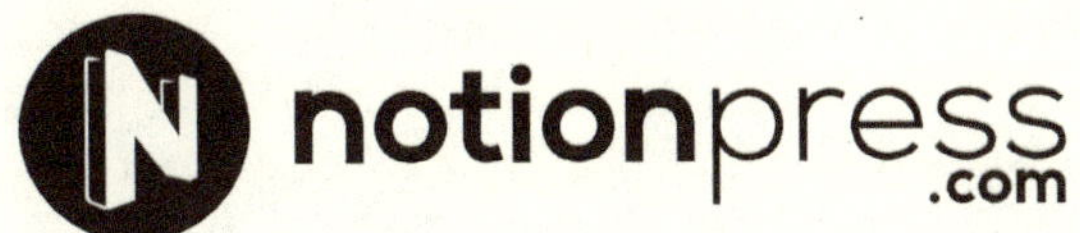

Notion Press

5 Muthu Kalathy Street, Triplicane,

Chennai - 600 005

First Published by Notion Press 2014

ISBN: 978-93-84381-63-9

This book is dedicated to

P. V. Narasimha Rao

(Patriotic statesman who believed that the nation is bigger than the political system)

Preface

Finally, An Indian author created an indispensable guide focuses on SAS Clinical Programming, in an instructive and conversational tone which helps them who want to make their career in SAS Clinical Programming and entry level programmers for their day to day tasks with practical, real world examples, detailed description, work flows, Issues, Resolutions, key techniques and many more.

This book is like your personal trainer, explains the art of SAS clinical Programming in 18 easy steps which covers from basics to ADS, TLF Creation, as well as CDISC SDTM, ADaM. Many statistical Concepts are explained in an easy way so that you feel confident while using Statistical Procedures. If you are already working as a SAS Clinical Programmer, still you need this book to sharpen your skills.

This book will be an asset to you and your career by making you a better SAS clinical Programmer.

Authors' Note

One interesting thing in SAS Clinical Programming, it is the career Option for people with various study backgrounds. I have seen SAS Programmers with different qualifications like Pharmacy, Statistics, M.C.A, M. Tech, M.Sc Life sciences, Bio Tech, Mathematics and many more. It is wonderful to see people with different backgrounds working on the same project, but how can we expect Clinical Research and Biostatistics knowledge from a person with technical qualification.

Every person might be strong in their own subject but SAS Clinical Programmer needs to know more than one subject (Programming (Tech), Clinical Research (Pharma) and Biostatistics (Stats)). This might be the reason I thought it would be beneficial to have a resource that brings together all these aspects in one volume so that it would help everybody who wants to make SAS Programming as their career Option.

This book was written to assist learners in getting started, while at the same time providing techniques that I have found to be useful to Entry level SAS Clinical programmers. This book is aimed more at the SAS Clinical programmer who is responsible for producing submission ready Reports.

This book assumes that the reader has no prior knowledge of clinical research and SAS programming. Each one of us has our own style of approach to an issue; it is likely that others will find alternate solutions for many of the issues discussed in this book.

The clinical trial data that appears in a number of examples throughout this book was just an imaginary phase 2 Diabetic study, any resemblance was simply accidental.

This book was organized in 18 easy steps from introduction to creating final reports, which resembles the SAS Clinical programmer's work environment.

The solutions to some of the questions are not written fully but only some steps of hints are mentioned. It is just for the sake of recalling the memory involving important facts in common practice.

I shall ever be thankful, grateful and eager to accept the insightful suggestions from my colleagues make this work more worthy.

Y L Prasad

Acknoweldgements

A great deal of information was received from the numerous people who offered their time. I would like to thank each and every person who helped me in creating this book.

I heartily express my gratitude to all of my peers, colleagues, friends and students whose sincere response geared up to meet the exigent way of expressing the contents. I am very much grateful to our Press, editors and designers whose scrupulous assistance completed this work to reach your hands.

Finally, I am personally indebted to my wonderful partner ***Prajwala***, and my kid ***Prakhyath***, for their support, enthusiasm, and tolerance, without which this book would have never been completed.

Y.L.Prasad

Contents

We all have dreams. But in order to make dreams
come into reality, it takes an awful
lot of determination, dedication,
self-discipline, and effort.

---Jesse Owens

STEP 1

INTRODUCTION TO CLINCAL RESEARCH

The Process from discovering a new drug to registering it for marketing is very complex and lengthy. There are several people involved in the Process of drug discovery and development includes Scientists, Clinicians, Statisticians as well as Data managers and SAS Programmers. It is estimated that, on average, a drug takes 10-12 years from initial research to reach the market. Drug discovery and development are mainly carried out by pharmaceutical companies and research agencies. The pharmaceutical market is very competitive. It is imperative that pharmaceutical companies discover and develop drugs efficiently and within the shortest time span to remain competitive.

Drug Development Process

The Drug development Process has different stages:

- Drug Discovery
- Drug Development
- Clinical Trials
- Manufacturing
- Marketing Approval

The Drug Discovery Process involves in finding out the target that causes the disease, chemical or biological compounds are screened and tested against these targets to find leading drug candidates for further development.

The Drug Development Process involves Tests performed on the lead compounds in test tubes (laboratory, in vitro) and on animals (in vivo) to check how they affect the biological systems.

The development Process includes pharmacological studies of the lead compound and its effects on toxicity, carcinogenicity, mutagenicity and reproductive development. These data are important for determining the safety and effectiveness of the lead compound as a potential drug.

Typically, tens of thousands of compounds are screened and tested, and only a handful makes it into the market as drug products. The statistics are such that, of 5000 compounds that show initial promise, five will go into human clinical trials, and only one will become an approved drug.

Clinical Research

Clinical research is a branch of healthcare science that determines the safety and effectiveness of medications, devices, diagnostic products and treatment regimens intended for human use.

Clinical research includes:

- ✦ Medical and behavioral research involving volunteer participants
- ✦ Investigations that are carefully developed and conducted with clinical outcomes recorded
- ✦ Identification of better ways to prevent, diagnoses, treats, and understands human disease
- ✦ Trials that test new treatments, clinical management and clinical outcomes, and long–term studies
- ✦ Strict scientific guidelines

There are ***ethical*** and ***regulatory constraints*** for the design and conduct of a clinical trial that have to be considered. Ethical principles are to protect participants before a drug is put forward for a clinical trial.

The United States National Institutes of Health (NIH) has stipulated seven ethical requirements:

1. Social value
2. Scientific validity
3. Fair subject selection
4. Informed consent
5. Favorable risk-benefit ratio

6. Independent review
7. Respect for human subjects

Clinical Trials:

Clinical trials are prospective studies on human subjects that are designed to answer specific questions about drugs, treatments, devices or new ways of using known interventions, generating ***safety*** and ***efficacy*** data.

Clinical Research is a study that tests how well an intervention works in a group of people, Tests for new methods of screening, prevention, diagnosis, or therapy. During a trial, additional information is learned about an intervention, its Risks, and its effectiveness.

Clinical Research Process

- Pre-clinical testing
- Investigational New Drug Application (IND)
- Phase I (assess safety)
- Phase II (test for effectiveness)
- Phase III (large-scale testing)
- Licensing (approval to use)
- Approval (available for prescription)
- Post-marketing studies (special studies and long-term effectiveness/ use)

Pre-Clinical Testing

Pre-clinical testing is required before testing humans. Pre-clinical testing is often conducted on animals many pre-clinical studies use a review Committee to determine if the use of animals is warranted. The review Committee also checks to see if the research can be improved by reducing or replacing animals. Laboratory and animal studies are conducted to find out if there is a potential benefit of the drug, vaccine, or other product and to explore general safety concerns. If a vaccine, Drug has a potential benefit, it is prepared for human testing. Pre-clinical testing takes approximately three to four years.

Investigational New Drug Application (IND):

For studies that involve a new vaccine, drug, after completing Pre-clinical testing, an investigational new drug application (IND) must be filed describing the results of pre-clinical testing and how future studies will be conducted. The U.S. Food and Drug Administration (FDA) have 30 days to review the IND. If the FDA approves the IND within 30 days, the test drug can precede to a phase I trial.

Phase I (Assess Drug Safety):

The Phase I clinical trial is the first experiment in which a drug is tested on the human body. The primary aim of the trial is to assess the safety of the new drug. Phase I trials are usually conducted with **open label**, i.e. the subjects are aware of the drugs that they are being given. For the first time, the Test drug is introduced to humans. Testing occurs in a small number of **healthy volunteers** (20 to 100). This initial phase of testing usually lasts several months to 1 year.

The goals of phase I clinical trials are Assess safety for humans as well as select the dose to be used in future studies. During phase I, the study is designed to determine how the human body reacts and what side effects occur as dosage levels is increased.

***Open-label Study**:* A trial in which subjects and investigators know which product each subject is receiving.

Phase II (Test for Safety and Effectiveness):-

A phase II study provides comparative information about relative safety and effectiveness and efficacy.

Most phase II studies are ***randomized*** trials. This means One group receives the experimental ***Test Drug*** other ***Control*** group receives the current standard treatment or ***Placebo***.

Some phase II studies are ***blinded***, This means participants and researchers do not know who receives the experimental test drug, this testing may last from several months to 2 years it may involve from 100-300 participants.

Phase III (Large-Scale Testing):-

The objective of Phase III is to confirm the efficacy of the drug in a large patient group. This trial is normally conducted in several hospitals in different demographic locations, to determine the influence of ethnic responses, so this trial is also known as a ***multicentre trial***. This large-scale testing (1,000-3,000 participants/volunteers) provides a better understanding of efficacy.

Most phase III studies are randomized and blinded trials with specific entry criteria. Phase III studies typically last several years. After a phase III study is successfully completed, a company can request ***NDA*** from the ***FDA***.

Randomization: The Process of assigning trial subjects to treatment or control groups using an element of chance to determine the assignments in order to reduce bias.

Blinded study: A study in which the subject, the investigator, or anyone assessing the outcome is unaware of the treatment assignment(s).

Control group: The group of subjects in a controlled study that receives no treatment, a standard treatment or a placebo.

Placebo: A pharmaceutical preparation that does not contain the investigational agent.

Multicenter trial: Clinical trial conducted according to a single protocol but at more than one site and therefore, carried out by more than one investigator.

Food and Drug Administration (FDA): The United States regulatory authority charged with, among other responsibilities, granting *IND* and *NDA* approvals.

New Drug Application (NDA): An application to FDA for a license to market a new drug in the United States.

Licensing (Approval to Use):

After all three clinical trial phases are complete and, if the research demonstrates that the test drug is safe and effective, a New Drug Application (NDA)/ Biologics License Application (BLA) is filed with the FDA. This NDA/BLA must contain all scientific information compiled over the course of the trials. The FDA is allowed at least 6 months to review the NDA/BLA. However, this review Process can sometimes take up to 2 years, depending on specific country requirements.

Approval (Available for Prescription):

Health care providers are able to prescribe. Even after approval, reviews continue to ensure safety over time. For example, all cases of adverse events must be reported, and quality control standards must be met (Sometimes studies to evaluate long-term effects are also required). The accelerated approval Process for serious diseases is designed to help development of treatments and to fill an unmet medical need to get important new treatments to patients faster.

Post-Marketing Studies:

Post-marketing studies (special studies and long-term effectiveness/ use) are also called **Phase IV** studies. These studies are often performed in special populations not previously studied (for example, children or the elderly) the studies are designed to monitor **Long-term** effectiveness and/or efficacy and the impact on a person's quality of life. Some studies help determine the cost -effectiveness of a therapy compared to other traditional and new therapies.

Industry Regulations and Standards for Clinical Trials

Every trial has to be approved and carried out under regulatory compliance to comply with GCP requirements. Different countries have different requirements for clinical trials. Two organizations that carry significant regulatory weight are the combined forces of the US Food and Drug Administration (***FDA***) and International Conference on Harmonization of Technical Requirements for Registration of Pharmaceuticals for Human Use ***(ICH***).

It is the role of public regulatory authorities to ensure that pharmaceutical companies comply with regulations. There is legislation that requires drugs to be developed, tested, trialed and manufactured in accordance to guidelines so that they are safe and patient's well being is protected.

Regulatory authorities perform the watchdog role to ensure that animal studies comply with Good Laboratory Practice (***GLP),*** clinical trials are performed in accordance with Good Clinical Practice (***GCP***) and drugs are manufactured under current Good Manufacturing Practice (***cGMP***) conditions.

ICH stands for "International Conference on Harmonization of Technical Requirements for Registration of Pharmaceuticals for

Human Use". ICH is a joint initiative involving both regulators and research-based industry representatives of the EU, Japan and the US in scientific and technical discussions of the testing Procedures required to assess and ensure the safety, quality and efficacy of medicines.

The objective of ICH is to increase international harmonization of technical requirements to ensure that safe, effective and high quality medicines are developed and registered in the most efficient and cost effective manner.

The ICH Topics are divided into four major categories:

- Quality (Q): Those relating to chemical and pharmaceutical Quality Assurance.
- Safety (S): Those relating to in vitro and in vivo pre clinical studies.
- ***Efficacy*** (E): Those relating to ***clinical studies*** in human subject.
- Multidisciplinary topics (M): Topics which do not fit uniquely into one of the above categories.

Efficacy Topics:

- ***E3: Structure and Content of Clinical Study Reports***
- E4: Dose-Response Information to Support Drug Registration
- ***E6: Good Clinical Practice: Consolidated Guideline***
- E8: General Considerations for Clinical Trials
- ***E9: Statistical Principles for Clinical Trials***
- E10: Choice of Control Group and Related Issues in Clinical Trials

ICH's mission is to make recommendations towards achieving greater harmonization in the interpretation and application of technical Guidelines and requirements for pharmaceutical product registration.

The ICH Steering Committee and its sub-committee are comprised of representatives from six parties that represent the regulatory bodies and research-based industry in the European Union, Japan and the USA.

Region	Regulatory Body	Research Based Industry
Japan	MHLW - Ministry of Health, Labour and Welfare	JPMA-Japan Pharmaceutical Manufacturers Association
Europe	EU - European Union	EFPIA - European Federation of Pharmaceutical Industries and Associations
USA	**FDA** - Food and Drug Administration	PhRMA - Pharmaceutical Research and Manufacturers of America

U.S.FDA: Branch of the United States Department of Health and Human Services and regulates all aspects of pharmaceutical industry.

21 CFR Part 11 Compliance: In your research the computer systems used to collect and analyze data must be validated to meet the FDA requirements for **electronic records and signatures.**

Title 21 of the Code of Federal Regulations (CFR):

Parts applicable to clinical research:

- Part 11 - Electronic Records and Signatures
- Part 50 - Protection of Human Subjects
- Part 54 - Financial Disclosure by Clinical Investigators
- Part 56 - Institutional Review Boards
- Part 312 - Investigational New Drug Application
- Part 314 - Applications for FDA Approval to Market a New Drug or an Antibiotic Drug
- Part 600 - Biological Products
- Part 812 - Medical Devices

Departments and Roles in a CRO

Contract Research Organization: *CRO* is an organization that provides support to the Pharmaceutical, biotechnology, and medical device industries in the form of research services outsourced on a contract basis. A *CRO* may provide such services as Pre Clinical Research, Clinical Research, Clinical Trials Management, Clinical Data Management, Bio statistics and SAS Programming.

A Typical Clinical Research Organization may contain the following departments:

- Clinical Operations
- Data Management
- Medical writing
- Pharmacovigilance
- Biostatistics/ SAS Programming
- Regulatory affairs

Key Functions in Clinical Operations:

- Managing and coordination of study conduct
- Monitoring and tracking of project milestones to ensure that the project runs within timelines.
- Participation as appropriate to expedite the feasibility and conduct of global trials
- Ensuring that the regulatory submission are of acceptable quality
- Support Investigator as and when required (e.g. Finalization of Investigator agreements and contracts, Finalization of ***Protocol*** and ***CRF***)

Key Functions in Data Management:

- Data Entry
- Database creation, Updating, Validation and Database lock
- Data Quality Check
- Data Clarification Form generation
- Coordination with Operations team to resolve queries

Protocol: Clinical research is conducted according to a plan (a protocol) or action plan. The plan describes what will be done in the study, how it will be conducted, and why each part of the study is necessary. The protocol or plan is carefully designed to safeguard the participant's health and answer specific research questions.

Case Report Form (CRF). A printed, optical, or electronic document designed to record all of the protocol-required information to be reported to the sponsor for each trial subject.

Key Functions in Quality Assurance:

- Facilitate audits which are conducted by clients locally within the country
- Ensure that all staff within the country has a complete and current training record
- Facilitate the auditing of suppliers and vendors used by company within the country
- Ensure that all *GCP* compliance issues with sites or elsewhere are raised to the Director of Quality Assurance and the Director of Medical Affairs
- Maintaining version control of ***SOP***s to ensure that all staff are following the correct and up to date *SOP*s

Key Functions in Pharmacovigilance:

- Collect, follow-up, transmit all local adverse events, and pregnancy cases, to Global Pharmacovigilance.
- Process cases in accordance with Global and Local Pharmacovigilance Procedures.
- Answer *ADR* and ***ADR*** case processing questions from local Regulatory Authorities and Health Care Professionals.
- Submit the report able *ADR*s, to the local Regulatory Authorities according to the national regulations and answer any subsequent questions in collaboration with the Global Pharmacovigilance.

Key Functions in Medical Writing:

- Clinical Study Protocol Writing
- Documentation for Regulatory Submission
- Technical Documentation for Clinical Trials
- Writing Medical Cases
- Managing ***SAE***s during clinical trials
- Closely associated with regulatory department in preparing narratives for submission

Standard Operating Procedure (SOP): Detailed, written instructions to achieve uniformity of the performance of a specific function.

Adverse Drug Reaction (ADR): Any noxious and unintended response associated with the use of a drug in humans.

Serious Adverse Event (SAE): Any untoward medical occurrence that at any dose: results in death, is life threatening, requires inpatient hospitalization or prolongation of existing hospitalization, results in persistent or significant disability/incapacity, or is a congenital anomaly / birth defect.

Process Flow in a Typical Clinical Trial

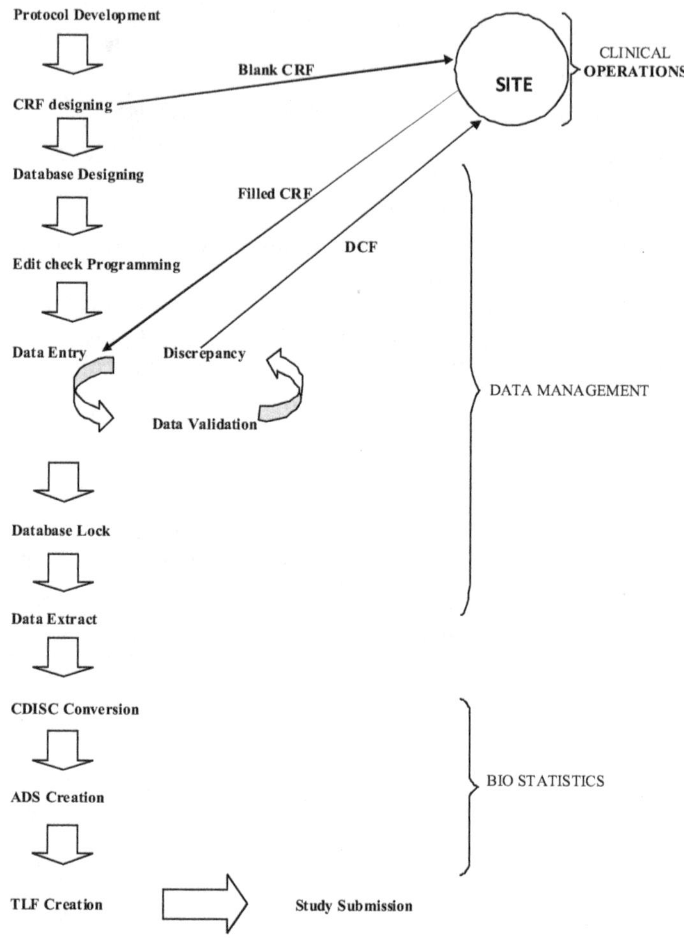

Process Flow in a Typical Clinical Trial:

Every clinical investigation begins with the development of a clinical protocol. The protocol is a document that describes how a clinical trial will be conducted and ensures the safety of the trial subjects and integrity of the data collected.

After preparing the protocol we go with CRF designing, The Case Report Form is a data-reporting document used in a clinical study. CRF Collects relevant data in a specific format in accordance with the protocol and compliance with regulatory requirements which

Allows efficient and complete data Processing, analysis and reporting and Facilitates the exchange of data across projects and organizations through standardization. CRF designer should always remember that Protocol determines what data should be collected on the CRF. All data must be collected on the CRF if specified in the protocol and Data that will not be analyzed should not appear on the CRF. CRF needs to be finalized and available before an investigator starts enrolling patients into a study. After designing and reviewing the CRF, it is a good idea to send them to sites that will be conducting the study and ask the site personnel for feedback.

Data collection is done using the CRF that may exist in the form of a paper or an electronic version. The traditional method is to employ paper CRFs to collect the data responses, which are translated to the database by means of data entry. These paper CRFs are filled up by the investigator according to the completion guidelines. In ***e-CRF*** method, chances of errors are less, and the resolution of discrepancies happens faster. The entries made in the CRF will be monitored for completeness and filled up CRFs are retrieved and handed over to the CDM team. CRF pages are entered by ***data entry*** operators. Best practice is, ***first pass data entry*** to be completed followed by a ***second pass*** or verification step by an independent operator.

Data validation is the Process of testing the validity of data in accordance with the protocol specifications. Edit check programs are written to identify the discrepancies in the entered data, which are embedded in the database, to ensure data validity. ***Discrepancy*** is defined as a data point that fails to pass a validation check. Discrepancy may be due to inconsistent data, missing data, range checks, and deviations from the protocol. If the data entered does not pass validation rules then a data query may be issued to the investigative site where the clinical trial is conducted to request clarification of the entry (***Data Clarification Form***). Any discrepancies between the first and second pass may be resolved such that the data entered is a true reflection of that recorded on the CRF. Where the operator is unable to read the entry the clinical data manager should be notified so that the entry may be clarified with the person who completed the ***CRF***. After a proper quality check and assurance, the final data validation is run. If there are no discrepancies, the SAS datasets are finalized in consultation with the statistician. All data management activities should have been completed prior to database lock. To ensure this, a pre-lock checklist is used and completion of all activities is confirmed. Once the approval for locking is obtained, the database is locked and clean data is extracted for statistical analysis. This data is often referred as raw data by SAS Programmers since this data is not ready for analysis. There may be many things to perform to convert the raw data to analysis ready data which is often refereed as ***ADS*** or ***VAD.*** Subsequent to ADS creation we go with ***TLF/*** Report generation followed by **CDISC** conversion and Submission.

STEP 2

INTRODUCTION TO SAS

SAS is a fourth-generation programming language. SAS is a comprehensive statistical software system which integrates utilities for ***Storing, Modifying, and Analyzing***, ***Graphing*** data. SAS is used in a wide range of industries such as Insurance, Education, Banking and Life sciences, etc.

Since SAS is a programming language, let us start by looking at a simple SAS program, such as this one:

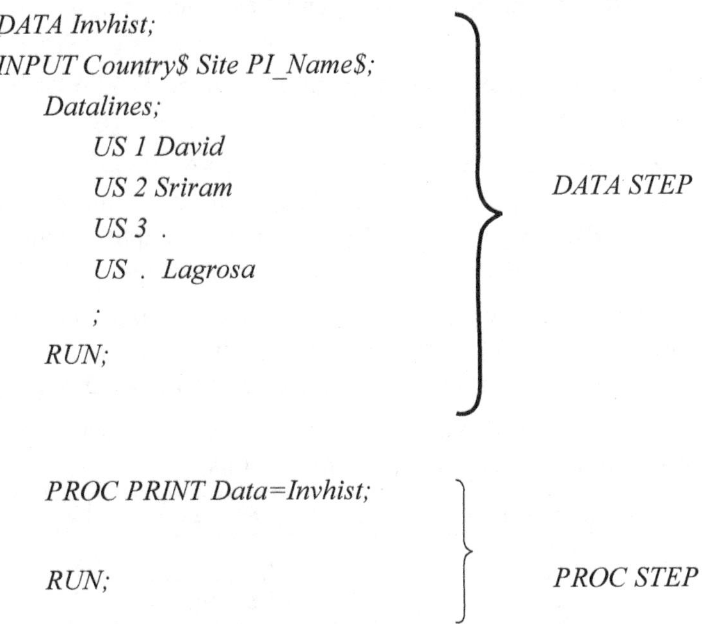

```
DATA Invhist;
INPUT Country$ Site PI_Name$;
    Datalines;
        US 1 David
        US 2 Sriram
        US 3 .
        US . Lagrosa
        ;
    RUN;

    PROC PRINT Data=Invhist;

    RUN;
```


SAS program is a *series of instructions* written in the SAS language that are executed in an order. We must adhere to a certain set of rules known as *SYNTAX*, in order for SAS to be able to read and run your programs properly.

Basic SAS Program Requirements:

- ✦ SAS statements typically begin with a SAS keyword and must end with a semicolon (;).
- ✦ SAS statements are not case sensitive, that is, they can be entered in any case.
- ✦ The words in SAS statements are separated by blanks or special character.
- ✦ Comments may be used to annotate your program. Two methods are:

  A delimited comment begins with a forward slash-asterisk (/*) and ends with an asterisk-forward slash (*/). All text within the delimiters is ignored by SAS.

  An alternative comment begins with an asterisk (*) and ends with a semicolon (;).

  All text between the asterisk (*) and the semicolon (;) is ignored by SAS.

SAS Program may contain one or more DATA or PROC steps or combination of both.

DATA steps are used to read data into a SAS data set, to modify data values, to check for and correct data errors, and to subset or merge data sets. **PROC steps** are used to calculate descriptive statistics, to generate summary reports, and to create summary graphs and charts.

SAS Datasets: In order to be able to analyze our data, we need to read it into a file that our SAS software understands. A SAS data set is a file containing two parts: a ***Descriptor portion*** and a ***Data portion***.

The data portion of a SAS data set is a collection of data values that are arranged in a rectangular table, such as this:

Country	Site	PI_Name
US	1	David
US	2	Sriram
US	3	
US	.	Lagrosa

SAS data set is comprised of variables and observations. The ***Variables*** (or columns) are collections of data values that describe a particular characteristic of the thing being measured. Our data set here contains just three variables — the Country, Site, and PI_Name. The ***Observations*** (or rows) are collections of data values that typically relate to one particular object.

Rules for User-Supplied SAS Names:

1. The first character must be a letter or underscore. Subsequent characters can be letters, numeric digits or underscores.
2. You can use upper or lowercase letters. SAS Processes names as uppercase regardless of how you type them.
3. Blanks cannot appear in SAS names.
4. When you create SAS data sets, do not use _NULL_, _DATA_, _LAST_.
5. Special characters, except for the underscore, are not allowed
6. All user supplied SAS names should be within the specified length.

SAS Variables:

There are two different types of Variables

1) Character: contain any value: letters, numbers, special characters, and blanks. Character values are stored with a length of 1 to 32,767 bytes. One byte equals one character.
2) Numeric: Stored as floating point numbers in 8 bytes of storage by default. Eight bytes of floating point storage provide space for 16 or 17 significant digits. You are not restricted to 8 digits.

The type of variable is just one of six variable attributes that SAS stores in the ***Descriptor portion*** of every SAS data set.

The six attributes that SAS stores are:

1) Variable Name
2) Variable Type
3) Variable Length
4) Variable Format
5) Variable Informat
6) Variable Label

SAS WINDOWS:

SAS is designed to be easy to use. It provides windows for accomplishing all the basic SAS tasks we need to do.

When we first open SAS (Windows O/S), by default, the five main SAS windows open:

- Program Editor or Editor Window,
- Log window
- Output window,
- Explorer window,
- Results window.

Editor window/ Program Editor: We can use either of these windows to enter, edit and submit SAS programs. The Program Editor window is available on all SAS platforms the (Enhanced) Editor Window, which is available only in the Windows operating environment.

For Windows operating systems, the default editor is called the Enhanced Editor, because it gives you a nudge — through the use of differently colored text.

Log window: The Log window displays messages about our SAS session and any SAS programs that we submit.

SAS uses the following color-coded system to assist you in reading the log:

Notes that SAS wants to report to you are printed in ***Blue***

Warnings that SAS wants to draw to your attention are printed in ***Green***

Errors that cause SAS to abort running your program are printed in ***Red***

(Info), DATA and PROC steps that appear in your program are printed in ***Black***

By default SAS Shows Errors, Warnings, Notes if your submitted program contains them, but ***Info*** would not be shown by default (By default Msglevel=N).

Output window: The Output window displays the output from SAS programs that we submit. It automatically opens or moves to the front of our display when we create output.

Explorer window: In the Explorer window, we can view and manage our SAS files and create shortcuts to files. Use this window to create new SAS libraries and SAS files, open any SAS file perform most file management tasks such as moving, copying, and deleting files.

Results window: The Results window helps us to navigate and manage output from SAS programs that we submit. We can view, save, and print individual items of output. The Results window is empty until we submit a SAS program that creates output.

Reading Data into a SAS Data Set:

In order to be able to analyze our data, we need to read it into a data set that our SAS software understands.

Prior to creating a dataset we need to ask ourselves the following questions:

1) ***Where our data reside:***
   - ✦ Are they in-stream data, that is, embedded within your SAS program?
   - ✦ Are they contained in a raw data file external to your SAS program?
   - ✦ Are they contained already in another SAS data set?
2) ***The format of the data***:
   - ✦ Are the data values arranged in neatly defined columns so that they can be read in using column input?
   - ✦ Are the data values separated by at least one blank space so that they can be read in using list input?
   - ✦ Do the data values contain special characters so that they must be read in using formatted input?
3) ***The kind of SAS data set that you want to create***:
   - ✦ Do you want to create a permanent SAS data set or temporary SAS data set?

If you want to create a permanent dataset you need to store the dataset in a ***permanent Library***.

Introduction to SAS/Library

A SAS data library is a collection of SAS files that are recognized as a unit by SAS on your operating Environment.

There are Libraries, which are been created by SAS at the time of Installation known as ***System defined*** (Work, Sashelp, and Sasuser etc) and We even can create libraries as per our requirement i.e. ***User defined*** Libraries.

Any System defined Library other than WORK and all used defined libraries are Permanent.

You can create libraries in two ways:

1. New library window Method
2. Libname statement

Rules for naming a libref:

- ✦ Must be 8 characters or less
- ✦ Must begin with a letter or underscore
- ✦ Remaining characters are letters, numbers, or underscores.

We can create SAS libraries using a point-and-click interface:

Click ***View → Explorer.*** Click ***File → New*** (New Library Window Opens), In the New Library window, specify information for the new library

- ✓ ***Name:*** Name of the Library (Libref)
- ✓ ***Engine:*** Default for Independent Library
- ✓ If you want the library to be created at the beginning of each SAS session, click Enable at startup check box.
- ✓ Provide the Path of the external folder by using browse button
- ✓ Click OK.

We can even create SAS libraries using LIBNAME Statement:

The LIBNAME statement establishes the library reference (or libref), which is an alias for the SAS data library. When you submit the LIBNAME statement, a connection is made between a libref in SAS and the physical location of files on your operating system.

Libname Libref Engine 'Path';

Creating a library by using libname statement:

Libname YLP 'E: \Clinitrial';

Where ***Libname*** → is the Keyword

YLP → Library Name (Libref),

E → is the Drive, ***Clinitrial*** → is Folder Name.

Libraries created by libname cannot be enabled but they are permanent.

The WORK library is the default library. If you do not specify a library reference on a SAS data set name, SAS assumes the libref is ***WORK***.

A work Library is gets deleted after the end of a SAS session and is not available for further Sessions. It is referenced by a ***one level name*** or with the first qualifier as ***WORK***.

A permanent library does not get deleted after a SAS session and is available all the time. It is referenced by a ***two level name.*** The first level name ***should not be*** WORK.

I don't look to jump over 7-foot bars: I look around for 1-foot bars that I can step over.

---Warren Buffett

STEP 3

INTRODUCTION TO OUR STUDY

Diabetes Mellitus:

Diabetes mellitus (**DM**) or simply diabetes is a group of metabolic diseases in which a person has high blood sugar. This high blood sugar produces the symptoms of frequent urination, increased thirst, and increased hunger. Untreated, diabetes can cause serious long term complications include heart disease, kidney failure, and damage to the eyes.

Diabetes is due to either the pancreas not producing enough insulin, or because cells of the body do not respond properly to the insulin that is produced.

Types of Diabetes Mellitus:

Type 1 DM results from the body's failure to produce insulin. This form was previously referred to as "insulin-dependent diabetes mellitus" (***IDDM***).

Type 2 DM results from ***insulin resistance,*** a condition in which cells fail to use insulin properly, sometimes also with an absolute insulin deficiency. This form was previously referred to as non insulin-dependent diabetes mellitus (***NIDDM***).

Gestational diabetes is the third main form and occurs when pregnant women without a previous diagnosis of diabetes develop a high blood glucose level.

Type 2 diabetes mellitus is the most common type characterized by ***insulin resistance***, which may be combined with relatively reduced insulin secretion. The defective responsiveness of body tissues to insulin is believed to involve the insulin ***receptor.***

The classic symptoms of untreated diabetes are weight loss, ***polyuria*** (frequent urination), ***polydipsia*** (increased thirst), and ***polyphagia*** (increased hunger).

Pathophysiology

Insulin is the principal hormone that regulates the uptake of glucose from the blood into most cells of the body, especially liver, muscle, and adipose tissue. Therefore, deficiency of insulin or the insensitivity of its receptors plays a central role in all forms of diabetes mellitus.

Insulin is released into the blood by ***beta cells*** (β-cells), found in the ***islets of Langerhans*** in the ***pancreas***, in response to rising levels of blood glucose, typically after eating, plays a critical role in balancing glucose levels in the body. Insulin can inhibit the breakdown of glycogen, it can stimulate the transport of glucose into fat and muscle cells, and it can stimulate the storage of glucose in the form of glycogen.

When the glucose concentration in the blood remains high over time, the kidneys will reach a threshold of reabsorption, and glucose will be excreted in the urine ***(glycosuria).*** This increases the osmotic pressure of the urine and inhibits reabsorption of water by the kidney, resulting in increased urine production (***polyuria***) and increased fluid loss. Lost blood volume will be replaced osmotically from water held in body cells and other body compartments causing dehydration and increased thirst (***polydipsia***)

Diagnosis:

Diabetes mellitus is characterized by recurrent or persistent hyperglycemia, and is diagnosed by demonstrating any one of the following.

- ***Fasting plasma glucose*** level ≥ 7.0 mmol/l (126 mg/dl).
- Plasma glucose ≥ 11.1 mmol/l (200 mg/dL) two hours after a 75 g oral glucose load as in a ***glucose tolerance test.***
- Symptoms of ***hyperglycemia*** and casual plasma glucose ≥ 11.1 mmol/l (200 mg/dl).
- Glycated hemoglobin (***HbA1C***) ≥ 6.5%.

WHO Diabetes diagnostic criteria:

Condition	2 hour glucose mmol/(mg/dl)	Fasting glucose mmol/(mg/dl)	HbA1c %
Normal	<7.8(<140)	<6.1 (<110)	<6.0
Impaired fasting glycaemia	<7.8(<140)	>=6.1(>=110)- <7.0(<126)	6.0 – 6.4
Impaired glucose tolerance	>=7.8 (>=140)	<7.0(<126)	6.0 – 6.4
Diabetes Mellitus	>11.1(>=200)	>=7.0(>=126)	>=6.5

Glucose production by the liver is normally maintained by a balance of the opposing actions of glucagon, which increases hepatic glucose release by stimulating gluconeogenesis and glycogenolysis, and insulin, which suppresses hepatic glucose release and promotes the storage of glucose as glycogen. Blockade of glucagon signaling through the glucagon receptor may be an effective approach to lower blood glucose in patients with type 2 diabetes mellitus (T2DM).

We planned our study with the assumption that our Test Drug reduces blood glucose by Blockade of glucagon signaling, and the details of study are follows.

STUDY DETAILS:

Title: *A Randomized, Double-Blind, Placebo-Controlled Phase 2 Study of Test Drug (CT1031975) in Patients with Type 2 Diabetes Mellitus.*

Objective: This Phase 2, multicenter, randomized, double-blind, Placebo -controlled, 4-arm, and parallel-group study examines the safety and efficacy of Test Drug (1, 3 and 6 mg) in patients with Type 2 diabetes

This Phase 2 study will further characterize the relationships between Test Drug dose and effects on measures of efficacy and hepatic safety.

The ***primary efficacy measure*** is the ***Mean HbA1c change*** from ***baseline to endpoint***

The ***primary safety measure*** of interest is the effect of Test Drug on the liver as assessed by ***liver function tests***.

The secondary objectives of the study are as follows:

To evaluate and compare the effects of Test Drug and placebo on blood glucose, glucagon, and glucagon-like peptide.

To evaluate the effects of Test Drug on patient perceptions of diabetes symptoms (for example, Cognitive, Hypoglycemic, Neuropathic, Psychological), as measured by the ***Diabetes Symptom Checklist-Revised*** (DSC-R).

To evaluate the effects of Test Drug on patient-reported satisfaction by means of the ***Perceptions about Medication-Diabetes*** (PAM-D) questionnaire.

Study Design:

This is an outpatient study. All study visits are to be conducted in the morning with the patient in the fasted state (at least 12 hours of fasting). Patients will sign an informed consent document (ICD) prior to screening at Visit 1. As soon as laboratory results have been received, eligible subjects may begin Visit 2. Visit 2 will begin the 1-week placebo lead-in period. At Visit 3, patients will be randomized to 1 of the 4 treatment groups.

Baseline measurements of safety and efficacy parameters will be made at Visit 3. After Visit 3, patients will return to the clinic at weekly intervals for the duration of the 12-week treatment period (Visits 4 through 15). For this study, the endpoint is defined as the end of the active treatment period, or Visit 15.

The Plan for Information to be collected from the subjects as follows:

Informed Consent Signed	- (V1)
Medical History	- (V1)
Physical Examination/ Height	- (V1)
Randomization	- (V3)
Blood Pressure/Heart Rate	- (V1 – V15)
Fasting Body Weight	- (V1 – V15)

Waist circumference	- (V1, V3, V15)
Fasting glucose	- (V1, V3 – V14)
Liver Function Tests	- (V1 – V15)
Adverse Events	- (V1 – V15)
Concomitant Medication	- (V1 – V15)
HbA1c	- (V1, V3, V5, V7, V9, V11, V13, V15)
Fasting Glucagon	- (V1, V3, V4, V5, V7, V9, V11, V13, V15)
Fasting GLP-1	- (V3, V4, V5, V7, V9, V11, V13)
DSC-R	- (V2, V3, V15)
PAM-D	- (V2, V3, V15)
OGTT (glucose, insulin, and C-peptide)	- (V3, V15)

Efficacy Measures:

Primary Efficacy Variable: The ***change in HbA1c***, from ***baseline to endpoint***, is the primary efficacy measure. Baseline is the Visit 3 HbA1c measurement. Endpoint will be the Visit 15 HbA1c measurement. If a patient discontinues before study completion, then the last observed HbA1c measurement post-randomization will be used as endpoint.

Secondary Efficacy Variables:

***Fasting Blood Glucose Concentration*:** Fasting blood glucose will be measured before randomization and before each protocol specified clinic visit. Change from baseline will be analyzed.

Fasting Insulin, Fasting Glucagon and Fasting GLP-1: Fasting insulin, glucagon and GLP-1 will be assessed at times outlined in the Study Schedule.

Patient sampling may occur concurrently with other analyte that are under investigation Safety variables:

Adverse Events (AE):

The incidence of treatment-emergent adverse events (***TEAE***) will be summarized by Medical Dictionary for Regulatory Activities (MedDRA) system organ class (SOC) and preferred term (PT), and overall. A TEAE is defined as an AE that first occurs or worsens (increases in severity) after baseline (Visit 3).

Serious Adverse Events (SAE):

The incidence of SAEs will be reported by MedDRA SOC and PT. Overall incidence rate of SAEs will be reported as well.

Adverse Events of Special Interest: The following are considered AEs of special interest:

- Elevated Lipase or Amylase
- Hypoglycemia
- Frequency counts and percentages of the events will be presented

Analysis Populations:

- The ***Intention-To-Treat*** (ITT) population is defined as all randomized patients.
- The ***modified ITT*** (mITT) population is defined as all randomized patients with at least 1 post baseline measurement and will be analyzed according to the treatment the patients were assigned.
- The ***Per-Protocol*** (PP) population is defined as all randomized patients who were compliant with study drug and completed the protocol.

Efficacy analyses (including the primary analysis) will be conducted on the modified ITT population.

Safety analyses will be performed on the population of randomized patients who receive at least one administration of study drug.

Flagging of Concomitant Medications as Prior, Prior and Concomitant or Concomitant:

- Medication start and stop dates will be compared to the date of first dose of study medication to allow medications to be classified as either Prior, Prior and Concomitant, or Concomitant.
- Medications that start and stop prior to the date of first dose of study medication will be classified as Prior medications.

- If a medication starts before the date of first dose of study medication and stops on or after the date of first dose of study medication then the medication will be classified as prior and concomitant.
- Medications will be classified as Concomitant if they have a start date on or after the date of first dose of study medication
- If medication start and/or stop dates are missing or partial, the dates will be compared as far as possible with the date of first dose of study medication.
- Medications will be assumed to be concomitant, unless there is clear evidence to suggest that the medication started prior to the first dose of study medication.
- If there is clear evidence to suggest that the medication started prior to the first dose of study medication, the medication will be assumed to be prior and concomitant, unless there is clear evidence to suggest that the medication stopped prior to the first dose of study medication.
- If there is clear evidence to suggest that the medication stopped prior to the first dose of study medication, the medication will be assumed to be prior.

Treatment Compliance:

Patient compliance with Test Drug will be assessed at each clinic visit. Acceptable compliance will be assumed if the study medication capsule count indicates that at least 80% of the assigned study medication was consumed

Baseline Definition:

Baseline is defined as the assessment at visit 3 (week 0). Change from baseline will be calculated as the visit value of interest minus the baseline value.

The first dose of study drug will be taken by the patient on the morning following visit 3. The first dose day will be referred to as study day 1.

Continuous data will be summarized in terms of the number of observations, mean, median, standard deviation, minimum and maximum.

Categorical data will be summarized in terms of the number of patients providing data at the relevant time point (n), frequency counts and percentages.

Efficacy Evaluation:

The primary efficacy endpoint is the mean change in HbA1c from baseline to endpoint. Baseline is defined as the HbA1c measurement at Visit 3 (Week 0).All HbA1c measurements up to and including Visit 15 (Week 12) will be used in the analysis.

A ***mixed-effects model for repeated measures*** (MMRM) will be used for the primary analysis. The model will consist of baseline HbA1c as a covariate, metformin use (yes/no), clinic visit, treatment, and clinic visit-by treatment interaction as fixed effects. The dependent variable will be the post baseline change from the baseline value.

Categorical analyses will be performed to compare the proportion of patients who achieve target HbA1c levels at Visit 15 by treatment group. A Cochran-Mantel-Hansel test will be used, stratified by baseline HbA1c.

Safety Evaluation:

- ✦ Extent of Exposure: Overall exposure to study drug will be calculated as the date of discontinuation from study treatment minus the date of first dose plus one. Overall exposure in weeks, calculated as the integer (ceiling) value of the difference defined above divided by 7, will be summarized using descriptive statistics.

Adverse Events

- ✦ Treatment-emergent adverse events will be tabulated i.e. those events which were not present at baseline or worsened in severity following the start of treatment.
- ✦ The onset date of an adverse event will be compared to the date of first dose of study medication to determine if the adverse event is treatment emergent or not.
- ✦ Adverse events with an onset date on or after the date of first dose of study medication will be classified as treatment emergent.

- If the adverse event onset date is missing or partial, the date will be compared as far as possible with the date of first dose of study medication.
- Adverse events will be assumed to be treatment-emergent, unless there is clear evidence to suggest that the adverse event started prior to the first dose of study medication.

Clinical Laboratory Evaluation: The numbers and percentages of patients who have abnormally low or abnormally high laboratory values will be provided by treatment group and by clinic visit.

STEP 4

STUDY DATASETS

Let us start with creating datasets which are useful for our study. (Often client may directly give you Datasets which are extracted from Database).

Dataset Invhist (Investigator History).

```
DATA YLP.Invhist (Label= Investigator History);
LENGTH Site 3 PI_Name $18 Country $ 3;
INPUT Country$ Site PI_Name$;
LABEL PI_Name = Principal Investigator Name
Site=Investigative Site
Country= Country;
Datalines;
USA 1 Mike_David
USA 2 Prasad_Sriram
USA 3 Ellis_Kimberley
USA 5 Lagrosa_Pedro
USA 6 Miller_David
USA 7 Wittmer_Bret
USA 8 Gaines_Marc
USA 9 Samson_Mercedes
;
Run;
```

- By submitting the above ***Data step*** we created a ***Dataset*** (Invhist) in ***permanent Library*** (YLP), the dataset has three (3) ***Variables*** and eight (8) ***Observations***. In the Input statement we simply listed the variable names leaving a space between name, this style is called ***List Input Style.***

> ***Investigator:*** is the individual designated to have the appropriate level of authority and responsibility to direct the research project.
>
> ***Site/Centre:*** is a location at which patients are recruited into clinical trials and to which patients return for ongoing review and treatment during the trial. A site may be a hospital or a research organization.
>
> ***Country:*** Country of the investigational site in which the subject participated in the trial.

List Input Method

List Input: In this method we simply list the variable names leaving at least one space between names in the order in which the variables appear in the data file.

Remember to use the ***dollar sign ($)*** to distinguish character variables from numeric variables.

This method is the easiest method to read the data but we must take note of the following restrictions:

- Fields must be separated by at least one blank (or other delimiter).
- Fields must be read in order from left to right.
- You cannot skip or re-read fields.
- Missing values must be represented by a place holder such as a period.
- Character values cannot contain embedded blanks.
- The default length of character values is 8 bytes. A longer value is truncated when it is written to the data set. (NOTE: 1 byte = 1 character).
- Data must be in standard character or numeric format.

Points to consider:

- ***Data statement*** begins the DATA step and names the data set that is being created.
- ***Length statement*** is used to assign length to each variable, otherwise by default SAS assigns length of 8 to each variable either character or numeric.
- ***Label statement*** is used to assign descriptive Labels to variable names. The order of the variables in the dataset is as mentioned in Label statement.
- The ***Datalines statement*** marks the beginning of the input data. The single semicolon marks the end of the input data and the DATA step.

Double Trailing AT Method (@@)

In this method we can ***read multiple observations per line of raw data***, we can use double trailing at signs (@@) at the end of your INPUT statement. This line hold specifier will hold that line of data, continuing to read observations until it reached end of the line.

DEMOGRAPHIC DATA: The characteristics of participant group or populations. This could include data on Race, Age, Sex and Medical history, all of which can be relevant to the clinical trial study findings.

Subject: A person who is the focus of scientific or medical attention or experiment. A subject in a clinical trial is not necessarily a patient, but a patient in a clinical trial is a subject.

Ethnicity: Denotes social groups with a shared history, sense of identity, geography and cultural roots.

Demographic Dataset:

Data YLP.Demog;

Length Patid 4 Site 3 Sex 3 Ethnic$ 3 Race 3 Birthyr 4;

Input Patid Site Sex Ethnic $ Race Birthyr @@;

Label Ethnic= Ethnic 0 - Not Hispanic or Latino 1 - Hispanic or Latino

Race= Race 1–White 2-Black 3-American Indian

Sex= Sex 1-Female 2–Male

Birthyr= Birth Year;

Datalines;

101 1 2 0 1 1958 **102** 1 . 1 1 1956 **103** 1 1 . 1 1955 **104** 1 1 0 1 1949 **105** 1 1 0 1 1941
201 2 1 1 1 1967 **202** 2 2 1 1 1962 **203** 2 2 0 2 1938 **204** 2 2 1 1 1952 **205** 2 2 1 1 1958
301 3 2 0 1 1955 **302** 3 2 0 2 1941 **303** 3 . 1 1 1969 **304** 3 1 0 1 1942 **305** 3 1 0 1 1959
501 5 1 0 1 1960 **502** 5 1 0 1 1955 **503** 5 1 0 2 1963 **504** 5 2 1 3 1952 **505** 5 2 1 3 1969
601 6 1 0 1 1939 **602** 6 1 1 3 1977 **603** 6 1 0 1 1944 **604** 6 2 0 1 1942 **605** 6 2 0 1 1947
701 7 1 0 1 1961 **702** 7 2 0 1 1945 **703** 7 1 0 1 1953 **704** 7 2 0 1 1947 **705** 7 1 0 1 1977
801 8 2 0 1 1942 **802** 8 2 0 2 1949 **803** 8 1 0 2 1957 **804** 8 2 0 2 1962 **805** 8 1 0 2 1960
901 9 2 0 2 1950 **902** 9 1 0 1 1943 **903** 9 1 1 1 1960 **904** 9 2 1 1 1960 **905** 9 1 0 1 1942

;

Run;

To make the Dataset Analysis ready we need to make the following modifications

- Demog dataset has Birthyr Variables which contains only Birth year, we need to ***Impute*** (Complete) the Birth date (As per SAP).
- ***Derive Ageyr*** Variable (As per Analysis Dataset Specifications)
- Create ***Age Group*** Variable (>65, <=65) (As per Mock shell)
- Create ***Flag Variables*** and group them as Subject Enrolled Set, Subject Completer Set, Subject Intent to Treat Set, Subject Modified Intent to Treat Set, Subject Per Protocol Set, Subject Safety Set, As per Analysis Populations mentioned in SAP.

Statistical Analysis Plan (SAP): A document that contains a more technical and detailed elaboration of the principal features of the analysis described in the protocol, and includes detailed Procedures for executing the statistical analysis of the primary and secondary variables and other data.

Analysis Dataset: An organized collection of data or information with a common theme arranged in rows and columns and represented as a single file, comparable to a database table.

Analysis Set: A set of subjects whose data are to be included in the main analyses. This should be defined in the statistical section of the protocol.

Analysis Variables: Variables used to test the statistical hypotheses identified in the protocol and analysis plan, variables to be analyzed.

Reading Non Standard Data (Format Input Method)

In this dataset ***Informed Consent Date*** is known as ***Non standard data***. Non standard data includes Dates, Numbers with embedded commas or dollar signs. To read non standard data we use informats.

There are three general types of informats:

- ✦ Character -- $InformatW.
- ✦ Numeric -- InformatW.D, InformatW.
- ✦ Date -- InformatW.

Here → $ indicates character informats, ***INFORMAT*** is the name of the informat, → W is the total width, and → D is the number of decimal places.

→The period is very important part of the informat name. Without a period, SAS may try to interpret the informat as a variable name.

In the dataset Variable ***ICDT*** (Informed Consent Date) is read using ***ddmmyy10.,*** which is a date informat, by this, SAS will convert conventional forms of dates into a number, the number of days since January 1, 1960. This number is referred to as a ***SAS date value***.

```
Data YLP.Consent;
Length Patid 4 Site 3 Icdt 8;
Input Patid Site Icdt mmddyy10. @@;
Label Patid= Subject Identifier
      Site= Investigative Site
      Icdt= Informed Consent Date;
Format Icdt Date9.;
Datalines;
101 1 7/13/2013 102 1 7/28/2013 103 1 8/26/2013 104 1 8/28/2013 105 1 9/4/2013
201 2 3/27/2013 202 2 3/30/2013 203 2 3/31/2013 204 2 4/1/2013 205 2 4/2/2013
301 3 5/4/2013  302 3 6/3/2013 303 3 6/24/2013 304 3 7/10/2013 501 5 4/7/2013
502 5 4/7/2013  503 5 4/8/2013  504 5 4/16/2013 505 5 4/29/2013 601 6 3/31/2013
602 6 4/22/2013 603 6 6/5/2013  604 6 6/10/2013 605 6 7/20/2013 701 7 3/31/2013
702 7 4/9/2013  703 7 4/13/2013 704 7 4/27/2013 705 7 4/30/2013 801 8 3/31/2013
802 8 3/31/2013 803 8 3/31/2013 804 8 4/6/2013 805 8 4/6/2013 901 9 4/8/2013
902 9 4/16/2013 903 9 4/17/2013 904 9 4/18/2013 905 9 4/25/2013
;
Run;
```

Note in the above Dataset Site 3 has only 4 subjects (subject 305 did not signed the Consent) and Site 4 could not able to recruit any subject.

Informed Consent is the Process of learning the key facts about a clinical trial before deciding whether or not to participate.

- By reading the dates in this way we can easily find the number of days between two dates by subtracting one from the other.
- Informats are used when reading in the non standard data and formats are used to write out values as per our requirement.

A few selected informats and formats include:

- DollarW.D →Includes dollar sign and commas
- PercentW.D →Writes the number as a percent
- W.D →Where w is the width and d the number of decimal places
- ZW.D → Writes leading zeros
- $CharW. →Writes standard character data preserving leading blanks

- $W. → Writes standard character data

The application of these formats to the data values on the left could produce the following results:

- 2345.678 → dollar9.2 → $2,345.68
- 0.6723 → percent8.2 → 67.23%
- -0.6723 → percent8.2 → (67.23%)
- 2345.678 → 10.2 → 2345.68
- 2345.678 → z10.3 → 002345.678

Randomization Dataset

Data YLP.Rand;

Length Patid 4 Trt $7 Trtcd 3;

Input Patid Trt $ Trtcd @@;

Label Patid = Subject Identifier Trt=Treatment Arm Trtcd= Treatment Code;

Datalines;

102 6mg 4 105 3mg 3 201 3mg 3 202 3mg 3 205 Placebo 1 301 1mg 2 502 6mg 4 503 1mg 2 504 3mg 3 505 Placebo 1 602 1mg 2 603 6mg 4 604 Placebo 1 701 3mg 3 704 Placebo 1 801 3mg 3 804 3mg 3 805 3mg 3 902 3mg 3 903 3mg 3 905 6mg 4

;

Run;

Note: Subjects 101,103,104,203,204 signed Consent but did not Randomized

> ***Arm:*** A planned sequence of elements, typically equivalent to a treatment group. This study involves a comparison of Test Drug (1, 3 and 6 mg/kg/day) and placebo administered orally once-daily.
>
> ***Randomization***: The Process of assigning trial subjects to treatment or control groups using an element of chance to determine the assignments in order to reduce bias.

In our study, Patients who meet all criteria for enrollment will be randomized to double-blind treatment at Visit 3 to any one of the treatment (1mg, 3mg, 6mg, Placebo).

Note: We can observe that only few subjects randomized from the subjects given Informed Consent. These Subjects are known as ITT Population as per our SAP (Statistical Analysis Plan)

VISIT Dataset

Data YLP.Visit;

Length Patid 4 Visid 3 Plwkenrl 3 Visdt 8;

Input Patid Visid Plwkenrl Visdt mmddyy10. @@;

Label Patid = Subject Identifier Visid= Visit Identifier

Plwkenrl=Planned Number of Weeks since Enrollment Visdt= Visit Date;

Format Visdt date9.;

Datalines;

```
101 1 . 7/13/2013    102 1 . 7/28/2013 102 2 . 8/4/2013 102 3 0 8/11/2013 102 4 1 8/18/2013
102 5 2 8/25/2013 102 6 3 9/1/2013  102 7 4 9/8/2013 102 8 5 9/15/2013 102 9 6 9/22/2013
102 10 7 9/29/2013 102 11 8 10/6/2013  102 12 9 10/13/2013 102 13 10 10/20/2013
102 14 11 10/27/2013 102 15 12 11/3/2013  102 16 13 11/10/2013  102 17 14 11/17/2013
102 18 15 12/1/2013  103 1 . 8/26/2013 104 1 . 8/28/2013 105 1 . 9/4/2013 105 2 . 9/21/2013
105 3 0 9/28/2013 105 4 1 10/5/2013 105 5 2 10/12/2013 105 6 3 10/19/2013
105 7 4 10/26/2013  105 8 5 11/2/2013 105 9 6 11/9/2013 105 10 7 11/16/2013
105 11 8 11/23/2013 105 12 9 11/30/2013 105 13 10 12/8/2013 105 14 11 12/14/2013
105 15 12 12/21/2013 105 16 13 12/30/2013  105 17 14 1/4/2010  105 18 15 1/18/2010
201 1 . 3/27/2013 201 2 . 4/8/2013    201 3 0 4/15/2013  201 4 1 4/22/2013 201 5 2 4/29/2013
201 6 3 5/6/2013 201 7 4 5/13/2013  201 8 5 5/20/2013   201 9 6 5/27/2013 201 10 7 6/3/2013
201 11 8 6/10/2013 201 12 9 6/17/2013 201 13 10 6/24/2013  201 14 11 6/30/2013
201 15 12 7/7/2013 201 16 13 7/15/2013  201 17 14 7/22/2013 201 18 15 8/11/2013
202 1 .  3/30/2013    202 2 . 4/10/2013   202 3 0 4/17/2013 202 4 1 4/24/2013  202 5 2
5/1/2013   202 6 3 5/8/2013 202 7 4 5/15/2013 202 8 5 5/22/2013  202 9 6 5/29/20132 02 10 7
6/5/2013   202 11 8 6/12/2013 202 12 9 6/19/2013 202 13 10 6/26/2013  202 14 11 7/1/2013
202 15 12 7/9/2013 202 16 13 7/17/2013 202 17 14 7/24/2013  202 18 15 8/7/2013
203 1 . 3/31/2013 204 1 . 4/1/2013    205 1 . 4/2/2013 205 2 . 4/9/2013   205 3 0 4/16/2013
205 4 1 4/23/2013 205 5 2 5/1/2013   205 6 3 5/7/2013   205 7 4 5/14/2013 205 8 5 5/21/2013
205 9 6 5/28/2013  205 10 7 6/5/2013 205 11 8 6/9/2013 205 12 9 6/18/2013
205 13 10 6/25/2013 205 14 11 7/1/2013   205 15 12 7/8/2013 205 16 13 7/16/2013
205 17 14 7/23/2013  205 18 15 8/6/2013
;
Run;
```

> ***Visit:*** *A clinical encounter that encompasses planned and unplanned trial interventions, Procedures, and assessments that may be performed on a subject.*

Our Study is an outpatient study. All study visits are to be conducted in the morning with the patient in the fasted state. Patients will sign an informed consent document (ICD) prior to screening at Visit 1.As soon as laboratory results have been received, eligible subjects may begin

Visit 2. Visit 2 will begin the 1-week placebo lead-in period, at Visit 3, patients will be randomized to 1 of the 4 treatment groups (Placebo, 1mg, 3mg, 6mg) .

Baseline measurements of safety and efficacy parameters will be made at Visit 3.After Visit 3, patients will return to the clinic at weekly intervals for the duration of the 12-week treatment period (Visits 4 through 15), for this study, the endpoint is defined as the end of the active treatment period, or Visit 15. After completing the 12-week treatment period, patients will return to the clinic at weeks 13, 14, and 16 (Visits 16, 17, and 18, respectively) during the post treatment washout period.

Study Treatment Dataset

```
Data YLP. Sdytrt;
Length Patid 4 Site 3 Visid 3 Sdydosedt 8;
Input Patid Site Visid Sdydosedt mmddyy10. @@;
Label Patid= Subject Identifier Visid=Visit Identifier
Sdydosedt = Study Treatment Dose Date;
Format Sdydosedt date9.;
Datalines;
102 1 3 8/11/2013   102 1 4 8/18/2013 102 1 5 8/25/2013 102 1 6 9/1/2013 102 1 7 9/8/2013
102 1 8 9/15/2013 102 1 9 9/22/2013 102 1 10 9/29/2013 102 1 11 10/6/2013
102 1 12 10/13/2013 102 1 13 10/20/2013 102 1 14 10/27/2013 102 1 15 11/3/2013
105 1 3 9/28/2013  105 1 4 10/5/2013  105 1 5 10/12/2013 105 1 6 10/19/2013
105 1 7 10/26/2013 105 1 8 11/2/2013 105 1 9 11/9/2013 105 1 10 11/16/2013
105 1 11 11/23/2013 105 1 12 11/30/2013 105 1 13 12/8/2013 105 1 14 12/14/2013
105 1 15 12/21/2013 201 2 3 4/15/2013 201 2 4 4/22/2013 201 2 5 4/29/2013  201 2 6 5/6/2013
201 2 7 5/13/2013  201 2 8 5/20/2013 201 2 9 5/27/2013  201 2 10 6/3/2013
201 2 11 6/10/2013  201 2 12 6/17/2013 201 2 13 6/24/2013  201 2 14 6/30/2013
201 2 15 7/7/2013 202 2 3 4/17/2013 202 2 4 4/24/2013  202 2 5 5/1/2013  202 2 6 5/8/2013
202 2 7 5/15/2013 202 2 8 5/22/2013  202 2 9 5/29/2013  202 2 10 6/5/2013 202 2 11 6/12/2013
202 2 12 6/19/2013 202 2 13 6/26/2013 202 2 14 7/1/2013 202 2 15 7/9/2013 205 2 3 4/16/2013
205 2 4 4/23/2013  205 2 5 5/1/2013   205 2 6 5/7/2013 205 2 7 5/14/2013  205 2 8 5/21/2013
205 2 9 5/28/2013  205 2 10 6/5/2013 205 2 11 6/9/2013  205 2 12 6/18/2013
205 2 13 6/25/2013  205 2 14 7/1/2013 205 2 15 7/8/2013
;
Run;
```

Column Input, Column Pointer Method

In this program to read Socterm, Pterm and Llterm we used column input method since each of the variable's values is found in the same place in the data line. ***Column input*** has several advantages over list input like spaces are not required between values, missing values can be left blank, character data can have embedded spaces, and you can skip unwanted variables. The other variables are read with ***column pointer at*** (@) method, by using column pointer at move to a particular column before reading data.

Data YLP.Events;

Length Patid 4 Llterm $16 Pterm $16 Socterm $28 Aestdt 8 Aeendt 8 Aesev $8;

Input Patid Aesev aerel aeout Socterm $ 11-36 Pterm $ 41-55 Llterm $57-70

@73 Aestdt mmddyy10. @85Aeendt mmddyy10. ;

Label Patid=Subject Identifier Socterm=System Organ Class

Pterm=Preferred Term Llterm=Lowest Level Term

Aestdt=Event Start Date Aeendt=Event End Date Aesev=Event Severity

Aerel= 0-No 1-Yes Aeout= 1-Recovered 3-NR 9-UNK;

Format Aestdt date9. Aeendt date9.;

Datalines;

101 1 0 3	*skin disorders*	*dry skin*	*dry skin*	*1/1/1962 .*	
101 1 0 3	*eye disorders*	*dry eye*	*dry eye*	*1/1/2002 .*	
101 1 0 3	*nervous system disorders*	*headache*	*headache*	*1/1/1975 .*	
102 1 0 3	*endocrine disorders*	*hypothyroidism*	*hypothyroidism*	*1/1/2001 .*	
102 1 0 3	*lymphatic system disorders*	*anaemia*	*anemia*	*1/1/1966 .*	
102 1 1 1	*gastrointestinal disorders*	*diarrhoea*	*diarrhea*	*8/12/2013*	*8/18/2013*
102 1 0 3	*cardiac disorders*	*tachycardia*	*tachycardia*	*9/29/2013*	*10/6/2013*
103 2 0 3	*skin disorders*	*dry skin*	*dry skin*	*1/1/1974 .*	
103 2 0 3	*musculoskeletal disorders*	*coccydynia*	*coccyalgia*	*8/14/2000 .*	
103 2 0 3	*immune system disorders*	*food allergy*	*peanut allergy*	*1/1/1974 .*	
104 1 0 3	*respiratory disorders*	*asthma*	*asthma*	*1/1/2001 .*	
104 1 0 3	*vascular disorders*	*hypertension*	*hypertension*	*1/1/1982 .*	
104 1 1 1	*gastrointestinal disorders*	*peptic ulcer*	*peptic ulcer*	*1/1/1974 .*	
104 1 1 1	*gastrointestinal disorders*	*diarrhoea*	*diarrhea*	*5/1/2013 .*	
104 1 0 9	*psychiatric disorders*	*depression*	*depression*	*1/1/2004 .*	
104 1 0 3	*musculoskeletal disorders*	*osteoporosis*	*osteoporosis*	*1/1/2006 .*	
105 1 0 3	*eye disorders*	*cataract*	*cataracts*	*1/1/2005 .*	
105 2 1 1	*gastrointestinal disorders*	*dysphagia*	*dysphagia*	*1/1/1989 .*	
105 1 1 1	*nervous system disorders*	*headache*	*headache*	*1/1/1989 .*	
105 1 0 3	*vascular disorders*	*hypertension*	*hypertension*	*1/1/1990 .*	

105 1 0 3	*cardiac disorders*	*bradycardia*	*bradycardia*	*4/7/2007 .*	
105 1 0 3	*cardiac disorders*	*angina pectoris*	*angina pectoris*	*1/1/2013 .*	
105 2 1 9	*musculoskeletal disorders*	*arthralgia*	*knee pain*	*1/1/1989 .*	
105 1 1 9	*psychiatric disorders*	*insomnia*	*insomnia*	*1/1/1992 .*	
201 1 0 3	*eye disorders*	*miosis*	*const.pupils*	*3/27/2013 .*	
201 1 0 3	*metabolism disorders*	*obesity*	*obesity*	*1/1/1999 .*	
202 2 0 3	*infections and infestations*	*ear infection*	*ear infection*	*5/2/2013*	*5/11/2013*
202 2 0 3	*respiratory disorders*	*pharynx pain*	*sore throat*	*5/2/2013 .*	*5/11/2013*
203 1 0 3	*immune system disorders*	*seasonal allergy*	*seasonal allergy*	*12/1/2008 .*	
204 1 0 3	*ear disorders*	*deafness*	*hearing loss*	*1/1/1989 .*	
204 1 0 3	*vascular disorders*	*hypertension*	*hypertension*	*4/10/2006 .*	
205 1 0 3	*metabolism disorders*	*obesity*	*obesity*	*4/2/2013 .*	
205 1 0 9	*infections and infestations*	*onychomycosis*	*fungal infection*	*4/2/2013 .*	
502 1 0 3	*metabolism disorders*	*obesity*	*obesity*	*1/1/2013 .*	
502 3 0 3	*general disorders*	*fatigue*	*fatigue*	*4/17/2013*	*8/11/2013*
502 2 0 1	*musculoskeletal disorders*	*pain*	*pain in calf*	*4/17/2013*	*8/11/2013*
502 1 0 3	*general disorders*	*fatigue*	*fatigue*	*4/17/2013 .*	
502 2 1 1	*eye disorders*	*vision blurred*	*blurred vision*	*4/17/2013 .*	
502 1 0 3	*general disorders*	*thirst*	*thirst*	*4/17/2013 .*	
502 1 1 1	*gastrointestinal disorders*	*constipation*	*constipation*	*4/17/2013*	*7/14/2013*
503 1 0 3	*metabolism disorders*	*obesity*	*obesity*	*1/1/2013 .*	

503 1 0 3	*general disorders*	*thirst*	*thirst*	*4/16/2013 .*	
503 1 0 3	*gastrointestinal disorders*	*dry mouth*	*dry mouth*	*4/16/2013 .*	
503 1 1 1	*general disorders*	*fatigue*	*fatigue*	*4/16/2013 .*	
503 1 0 3	*general disorders*	*irritability*	*irritability*	*4/16/2013 .*	
504 1 0 3	*general disorders*	*thirst*	*thirst*	*4/23/2013 .*	
504 1 0 3	*nervous system disorders*	*paraesthesia*	*abnormal touch*	*4/23/2013 .*	
504 2 0 9	*musculoskeletal disorders*	*muscle spasms*	*muscle cramps*	*4/23/2013 .*	
504 2 0 3	*musculoskeletal disorders*	*myalgia*	*muscle soreness*	*4/23/2013 .*	
504 1 0 9	*nervous system disorders*	*burning sense*	*burning leg*	*5/1/2013 .*	
;					
Run;					

Adverse Event: An adverse event can be any unintended sign (including an abnormal laboratory finding), symptom, or disease temporally associated with the use of investigational product, whether or not related to the investigational product.

While Creating Analysis ready Datasets, we need to create the following Flag Variables:

- Event Identifier
- Visit Forward Identifier
- Event Sequence Identifier
- Treatment-Emergent AE Flag
- Event Continuing Flag

Column Pointer At Method

```
Data YLP . Cmtpy;

Length Patid 3 Visid 3 cmname $20 cmterm $20 cmdose 4 cmdoseu $4
Cmstdt 8 Cmendt 8 Cmfreq 3 Cmifu 3;

Input Patid @5 cmdose 4. @9 cmdoseu $4. @13 cmstdt mmddyy10.
@25 cmendt mmddyy10. @37 cmfreq    @41 cmname $20. @61
cmterm $20. @85 Visid  Cmifu;

Label Patid= Subject Identifier Visid= Visit Identifier

Cmdose=Therapy Dose

Cmdoseu=Therapy Dose UOM  Cmstdt=Therapy Start Date

Cmendt= Therapy End Date Cmname=Therapy Name

Cmterm= Therapy Dictionary Term

Cmfreq=Therapy Frequency 2- QD 4-BID 8-SOS

Cmifu= Indication for Use 4-AE 2-Prophylaxis 1-Study;
```

```
Format Cmstdt date9. Cmendt date9.;
Datalines;
101   440   mg    1/1/2003               8   aleve          naproxen        1 4
101   2     drop  1/1/2005               8   renu           renu            1 4
102   100   ug    6/1/2006               2   synthroid      levothyroxine   1 4
102   500   mg    7/25/2009              2   niaspan        nicotinic_acid  1 4
102   1     u     1/1/1988               2   multivitamin   multivitamins   1 2
102   1     u     1/1/2007               2   fibercon       polycarbophil   1 2
102   2000  mg    7/1/2008               4   metformin      metformin       1 1
103   20    mg    2/1/2013               2   lovastatin     lovastatin      1 4
103   2000  mg    1/1/2008               3   omega iii      fish oil        1 2
103   800   mg    1/1/2000               8   ibuprofen      ibuprofen       1 4
103   1000  mg    4/1/2013               4   metformin      metformin       1 1
104   2000  mg    4/25/2009              4   metformin      metformin       1 1
104   15    mg    1/1/2006               2   mobic          meloxicam       1 4
104   300   mg    1/1/2006               9   neurontin      gabapentin      1 4
105   2000  mg    1/1/2005               4   metformin      metformin       1 1
105   100   mg    1/1/1990               2   atenolol       atenolol        1 4
105   81    mg    1/1/2013               2   aspirin        acetylsalicylic 1 2
105   20    mg    1/1/2007               2   simvastatin    simvastatin     1 5
105   1     u     1/1/1999               2   multivitamin   multivitamins   1 2
105   1.3   mg    5/1/2007               8   albuterol      salbutamol      2 4
105   120   mg    1/1/1999               2   ginko biloba   ginkgo biloba   2 2
105   1000  mg    1/1/1999               2   vitamin c      ascorbic acid   2 2
201   1000  mg    1/1/2006               4   metformin      metformin       1 1
202   325   mg    5/2/2013    5/11/2013  8   acetaminophen  paracetamol     6 4
202   5     mg    5/2/2013    5/11/2013  8   phenylephrine  phenylephrine   6 4
202   500   mg    5/2/2013    5/11/2013  8   tylenol        paracetamol     6 4
203   500   mg    4/1/2008               4   metformin      metformin       1 1
204   500   mg    12/3/2003              4   metformin      metformin       1 1
204   20    mg    4/10/2006              2   crestor        rosuvastatin    1 4
204   5     mg    4/10/2006              2   lisinopril     lisinopril      1 4
205   180   mg    1/1/2007               8   allegra        fexofenadine    1 4
205   20    mg    5/23/2013   5/23/2013  2   nexium         esomeprazole    9 4
205   500   mg    7/10/2013              8   tylenol        paracetamol     16 4
301   325   mg    1/1/1965               8   aspirin        acetylsalicylic 1 2
301   200   mg    1/1/2000               8   naproxen       naproxen        1 2
302   1.2   g     9/1/2008               2   lialda         mesalazine      1 4
303   2000  mg    11/1/2008              4   metformin      metformin       1 1
304   20    mg    6/5/2013               2   lisinopril     lisinopril      1 4
501   500   mg    1/1/2002               4   metformin      metformin       1 1
503   500   mg    11/1/2007              4   metformin      metformin       1 1
504   500   mg    1/1/2007               5   metformin      metformin       1 1
505   500   mg    3/1/2004               4   metformin      metformin       1 1
505   40    mg    1/1/2007               2   lovastatin     lovastatin      1 4
;
Run;
```

Concomitant medication (con-med): is a drug or biological product, other than a study drug, taken by a subject during a clinical trial.

Dose denotes a quantity of a medication prescribed to be taken at one time or at stated intervals.

Unit is the term used to denote its amount. The metric system, e.g., mg, kg, mcg, ml is generally used. Other systems such as the ***international unit (IU)*** may be used as well. The international unit is a unit of measurement in pharmacology for the amount of a substance, based on measured biological activity. It is used for vitamins, hormones, some drugs, vaccines, and blood products.

Start/Stop date of a medication is the timeframe in which the medication was or is being used.

We need to create the following Variables in CMADS:

- Concomitant Therapy Identifier
- Treatment Type
- Therapy Continuing Flag

Data YLP.Labs;

Length Patid 4 Visid 3 LbProc $4 Lbtest $15 Lbdt 8 Lbrn 8 Lbru $ 8; Input Patid @5 Visid @9 LbProc$4. @13 Lbdt mmddyy10. @25 Lbnrhi @33 Lbnrlo @41 Lbrn @49 Lbru $ @57 Lbtest $;

Label Patid=Subject Identifier Visid= Visit Identifier

LbProc = Lab Procedure Lbdt= Lab Date Lbnrlo=Lab Normal Low Range

lbnrhi=Lab Normal High Range Lbrn=Lab Result Numeric

Lbru= Lab Result Unit Lbtest= Lab Test;

Format Lbdt date9.;

Datalines;

```
201  1  hem   3/27/2013  48    34    41      percent  hematocrit
201  1  hem   3/27/2013  16.4  11.6  13      gm/dl    hemoglobin
201  1  hem   3/27/2013  6.1   4.3   6.5     percent  hemoglobin_a1c
201  1  chem  4/7/2013   214   45    84.14   mg/dl    triglycerides
201  1  chem  4/7/2013   174   74    124.90  mg/dl    ldl_cholesterol
201  1  chem  4/7/2013   88    34    63.03   mg/dl    hdl_cholesterol
201  3  hem   4/15/2013  48    34    38      percent  hematocrit
201  3  hem   4/15/2013  16.4  11.6  12.7    gm/dl    hemoglobin
201  3  hem   4/15/2013  6.1   4.3   8.02    percent  hemoglobin_a1c
201  3  chem  4/15/2013  214   45    71.74   mg/dl    triglycerides
201  3  chem  4/15/2013  174   74    109.04  mg/dl    ldl_cholesterol
201  3  chem  4/15/2013  88    34    51.04   mg/dl    hdl_cholesterol
201  7  hem   5/13/2013  48    34    41      percent  hematocrit
201  7  hem   5/13/2013  16.4  11.6  13.3    gm/dl    hemoglobin
201  7  hem   5/13/2013  6.1   4.3   6.33    percent  hemoglobin_a1c
201  7  chem  5/13/2013  214   45    83.25   mg/dl    triglycerides
201  7  chem  5/13/2013  174   74    131.86  mg/dl    ldl_cholesterol
```

```
201  7   chem  5/13/2013  88    34    61.09   mg/dl    hdl_cholesterol
201  11  hem   6/10/2013  48    34    43      percent  hematocrit
201  11  hem   6/10/2013  16.4  11.6  13.1    gm/dl    hemoglobin
201  11  hem   6/10/2013  6.1   4.3   4.86    percent  hemoglobin_a1c
201  11  chem  6/10/2013  214   45    100.97  mg/dl    triglycerides
201  11  chem  6/10/2013  174   74    119.10  mg/dl    ldl_cholesterol
201  11  chem  6/10/2013  88    34    68.05   mg/dl    hdl_cholesterol
202  1   hem   3/30/2013  54    39    49      percent  hematocrit
202  1   hem   3/30/2013  18.1  12.7  16.1    gm/dl    hemoglobin
202  1   hem   3/30/2013  6.1   4.3   9       percent  hemoglobin_a1c
202  1   chem  4/10/2013  327   55    161.20  mg/dl    triglycerides
202  1   chem  4/10/2013  202   97    93.96   mg/dl    ldl_cholesterol
202  1   chem  4/10/2013  64    30    42.15   mg/dl    hdl_cholesterol
202  3   hem   4/17/2013  54    39    48      percent  hematocrit
202  3   hem   4/17/2013  18.1  12.7  16.4    gm/dl    hemoglobin
202  3   hem   4/17/2013  6.1   4.3   6.62    percent  hemoglobin_a1c
202  3   chem  4/17/2013  327   55    185.11  mg/dl    triglycerides
202  3   chem  4/17/2013  202   97    95.12   mg/dl    ldl_cholesterol
202  3   chem  4/17/2013  64    30    42.15   mg/dl    hdl_cholesterol
202  7   hem   5/15/2013  54    39    43      percent  hematocrit
202  7   hem   5/15/2013  18.1  12.7  14.3    gm/dl    hemoglobin
202  7   hem   5/15/2013  6.1   4.3   3.70    percent  hemoglobin a1c
202  7   chem  5/15/2013  327   55    176.26  mg/dl    triglycerides
202  7   chem  5/15/2013  202   97    73.85   mg/dl    ldl_cholesterol
202  7   chem  5/15/2013  64    30    37.89   mg/dl    hdl_cholesterol
202  11  hem   6/12/2013  54    39    46      percent  hematocrit
202  11  hem   6/12/2013  18.1  12.7  15.8    gm/dl    hemoglobin
202  11  hem   6/12/2013  6.1   4.3   5.48    percent  hemoglobin_a1c
202  11  chem  6/12/2013  327   55    167.40  mg/dl    triglycerides
202  11  chem  6/12/2013  202   97    87.00   mg/dl    ldl_cholesterol
202  11  chem  6/12/2013  64    30    47.17   mg/dl    hdl_cholesterol
;
Run;
```

While Creating LBADS or ADLB Datasets, we need to create the following Variables:

- Lab Sequence Number
- Age at Lab Collection
- Lab Test Normality
- Lab Imputation Flag
- Baseline Flag
- Baseline Value
- Change from Baseline to Visit
- Change from Previous Visit
- Endpoint Flag
- Percent Change Baseline to Visit
- Percent Change from Previous Visit

Vital signs are measures of various physiological statistics, often taken to assess the most basic body function. Vital signs normally record body temperature, pulse rate (or heart rate), blood pressure, and respiratory rate, but may also include other measurements.

```
Data YLP.Vitals;
Length Patid 4 Visid 3 Vstest $4 Vsrn 4 Vsdt 8 Vsru$ 5;
Input Patid @5 Visid @9 Vstest$ @13 Vsrn @17 Vsdt mmddyy10. @29
Vsru ;
Label Patid = Subject Identifier  Visid=Visit Identifier
Vstest=Vital Sign Name  Vsrn=Vital Sign Result Numeric
Vsdt=Vital Sign Date        Vsru=Vital Sign Result unit;
Format vsdt date9.;
```

Datalines;

```
201 1 hgt 168 3/27/2013 cm 201 1 wc 121 7/7/2013 cm
201 1 wgt 114 3/27/2013 kg 201 1 hrt 58 3/27/2013 bpm
201 2 hrt 61 4/8/2013 bpm 201 3 hrt 58 4/15/2013 bpm
201 4 hrt 62 4/22/2013 bpm 201 5 hrt 59 4/29/2013 bpm
201 6 hrt 60 5/6/2013 bpm 201 7 hrt 60 5/13/2013 bpm
201 8 hrt 57 5/20/2013 bpm 201 9 hrt 62 5/27/2013 bpm
201 10 hrt 60 6/3/2013 bpm 201 11 hrt 59 6/10/2013 bpm
201 12 hrt 64 6/17/2013 bpm 201 13hrt 59 6/24/2013 bpm
201 14 hrt 61 6/30/2013 bpm 201 15 hrt 60 7/7/2013 bpm
201 16 hrt 59 7/15/2013 bpm 201 17 hrt 57 7/22/2013 bpm
201 18 hrt 55 8/11/2013 bpm 201 1 dia 74 3/27/2013 mmHg
201 2 dia 72 4/8/2013 mmHg 201 3 dia 70 4/15/2013 mmHg
201 4 dia 69 4/22/2013 mmHg 201 5 dia 76 4/29/2013 mmHg
201 6 dia 70 5/6/2013 mmHg 201 7 dia 72 5/13/2013 mmHg
201 8 dia 69 5/20/2013 mmHg 201 9 dia 60 5/27/2013 mmHg
201 10 dia 66 6/3/2013 mmHg 201 11 dia 66 6/10/2013 mmHg
201 12 dia 74 6/17/2013 mmHg 201 13 dia 61 6/24/2013 mmHg
201 14 dia 67 6/30/2013 mmHg 201 15 dia 76 7/7/2013 mmHg
201 16 dia 68 7/15/2013 mmHg 201 17 dia 68 7/22/2013 mmHg
201 18 dia 67 8/11/2013 mmHg 201 1 sys 118 3/27/2013 mmHg
201 2 sys 116 4/8/2013 mmHg 201 3 sys 122 4/15/2013 mmHg
201 4 sys 101 4/22/2013 mmHg 201 5 sys 119 4/29/2013 mmHg
201 6 sys 126 5/6/2013 mmHg 201 7 sys 123 5/13/2013 mmHg
201 8 sys 92 5/20/2013 mmHg 201 9 sys 112 5/27/2013 mmHg
201 10 sys 115 6/3/2013 mmHg 201 11 sys 117 6/10/2013 mmHg
201 12 sys 115 6/17/2013 mmHg 201 13 sys 113 6/24/2013 mmHg
201 14 sys 115 6/30/2013 mmHg 201 15 sys 116 7/7/2013 mmHg
201 16 sys 112 7/15/2013 mmHg 201 17 sys 116 7/22/2013 mmHg
201 18 sys 108 8/11/2013 mmHg 202 1 wc 92 7/9/2013 cm
202 1 wgt 70 3/30/2013 kg 202 1 hgt 164 3/30/2013 cm
202 1 hrt 68 3/30/2013 bpm 202 2 hrt 68 4/10/2013 bpm
202 3 hrt 78 4/17/2013 bpm 202 4 hrt 70 4/24/2013 bpm
202 5 hrt 79 5/1/2013 bpm 202 6 hrt 66 5/8/2013 bpm
202 7 hrt 69 5/15/2013 bpm 202 8 hrt 76 5/22/2013 bpm
202 9 hrt 70 5/29/2013 bpm 202 10 hrt 74 6/5/2013 bpm
202 11 hrt 70 6/12/2013 bpm 202 12 hrt 66 6/19/2013 bpm
202 13 hrt 72 6/26/2013 bpm 202 14 hrt 78 7/1/2013 bpm
202 15 hrt 75 7/9/2013 bpm 202 16 hrt 73 7/17/2013 bpm
202 17 hrt 80 7/24/2013 bpm 202 18 hrt 78 8/7/2013 bpm
202 1 dia 88 3/30/2013 mmHg 202 2 dia 88 4/10/2013 mmHg
202 3 dia 78 4/17/2013 mmHg 202 4 dia 88 4/24/2013 mmHg
202 5 dia 84 5/1/2013 mmHg 202 6 dia 72 5/8/2013 mmHg
202 7 dia 82 5/15/2013 mmHg 202 8 dia 80 5/22/2013 mmHg
202 9 dia 84 5/29/2013 mmHg 202 10 dia 89 6/5/2013 mmHg
```

```
202 11 dia 90 6/12/2013 mmHg 202 12 dia 82 6/19/2013 mmHg
202 13 dia 86 6/26/2013 mmHg 202 14 dia 86 7/1/2013 mmHg
202 15 dia 88 7/9/2013 mmHg 202 16 dia 89 7/17/2013 mmHg
202 17 dia 85 7/24/2013 mmHg 202 18 dia 91 8/7/2013 mmHg
202 1 sys 130 3/30/2013 mmHg 202 2 sys 148 4/10/2013 mmHg
202 3 sys 124 4/17/2013 mmHg 202 4 sys 133 4/24/2013 mmHg
202 5 sys 130 5/1/2013 mmHg 202 6 sys 113 5/8/2013 mmHg
202 7 sys 124 5/15/2013 mmHg 202 8 sys 118 5/22/2013 mmHg
202 9 sys 136 5/29/2013 mmHg 202 10 sys 140 6/5/2013 mmHg
202 11 sys 125 6/12/2013 mmHg 202 12 sys 111 6/19/2013 mmHg
202 13 sys 134 6/26/2013 mmHg 202 14 sys 132 7/1/2013 mmHg
202 15 sys 133 7/9/2013 mmHg 202 16 sys 134 7/17/2013 mmHg
202 17 sys 129 7/24/2013 mmHg 202 18 sys 125 8/7/2013 mmHg
;
Run;
```

While Creating VSADS or ADVS Datasets, we need to create the following Variables:

- *Vital* Sign Sequence Identifier
- Original Result Flag
- Baseline Flag - TR Phase
- Baseline Value - TR Phase
- Change from Baseline to Visit - TR Phase
- Change from Previous Visit - TR Phase
- Endpoint Flag - TR Phase
- Pct Chg Baseline to Visit - TR Phase
- Pct Chg from Previous Visit - TR Phase

```
Data YLP.Disposit;
Input Patid 4. @5 Invid @9 Ds @13 Dssnm $40. @53 Visid @57 Dsdt mmddyy10. @69 Dscom $12.;
Format Dsdt Date9.;
Datalines;
101 1 5 Inclusion/Exclusion Criteria not met 1 7/13/2013 Exclusion 27
103 1 5 Inclusion/Exclusion Criteria not met 1 8/26/2013 Exclusion 15
104 1 5 Inclusion/Exclusion Criteria not met 1 8/28/2013 Inclusion 06
201 2 1 Completed 18 8/11/2013.
202 2 1 Completed 18 8/7/2013.
203 2 5 Inclusion/Exclusion Criteria not met 1 3/31/2013 Exclusion 18
204 2 5 Inclusion/Exclusion Criteria not met 1 4/1/2013 Inclusion 07
205 2 1 Completed 18 8/6/2013.
301 3 4 Lost to follow up 5 6/2/2013 Sent letter
302 3 5 Inclusion/Exclusion Criteria not met 1 6/3/2013 Inclusion 06
303 3 5 Inclusion/Exclusion Criteria not met 1 6/24/2013 Inclusion 06
304 3 5 Inclusion/Exclusion Criteria not met 1 7/10/2013 Inclusion 06
501 5 5 Inclusion/Exclusion Criteria not met 1 4/7/2013 Inclusion 03
502 5 1 Completed 18 8/11/2013.
503 5 1 Completed 18 8/12/2013.
504 5 2 Adverse Event 4 5/8/2013.
505 5 5 Inclusion/Exclusion Criteria not met 1 4/29/2013 Inclusion 06
601 6 5 Inclusion/Exclusion Criteria not met 1 4/1/2013 Inclusion 06
602 6 1 Completed 18 9/1/2013.
603 6 1 Completed 18 10/6/2013.
604 6 5 Inclusion/Exclusion Criteria not met 1 6/10/2013 Inclusion 05
605 6 5 Inclusion/Exclusion Criteria not met 1 7/20/2013 Exclusion 24
701 7 1 Completed 18 8/10/2013.
702 7 5 Inclusion/Exclusion Criteria not met 1 4/9/2013 Exclusion 15
703 7 5 Inclusion/Exclusion Criteria not met 1 4/13/2013 Inclusion 06
704 7 7 Subject Decision . 8/4/2013 Sub refused.
705 7 7 Subject Decision 1 4/30/2013 Not able.
801 8 6 Protocol Violation . 6/24/2013 On_fibrate.
802 8 5 Inclusion/Exclusion Criteria not met 1 3/31/2013 Exclusion 21
803 8 5 Inclusion/Exclusion Criteria not met 1 3/31/2013 Inclusion 06
```

```
804 8 7 Subject Decision                          10 6/8/2013   withdrew_IC
805 8 1 Completed                                 18 8/10/2013.
901 9 5 Inclusion/Exclusion Criteria not met      1  4/8/2013   Inclusion 06
902 9 4 Lost to follow up                         5  5/27/2013  Legal_Issue
903 9 1 Completed                                 18 8/27/2013.
904 9 5 Inclusion/Exclusion Criteria not met      1  4/18/2013  Inclusion 06
905 9 1 Completed                                 18 9/3/2013.
;
Run;
```

```
Data YLP. Effdiab;
Input Patid Visid HbA1c_rn Fsg_rn Fgluc_rn Fglp_rn  Wgt_rn @@;
Label Patid=Subject Identifier Visid=Visit Identifier
Hba1c_rn= Hemoglobin A1C Result Numeric (%)
Fsg_rn=Fasting Serum Glucose Result Numeric (mg/dL)
Fgluc_rn= Fasting Glucagon Result (pmol/L)
Fglp1_rn= Fasting GLP-1 Result (pmol/L)
Wgt_rn=Weight Result Numeric (kg);
```

Datalines;

```
101 1 12.6 215.25 . . 123 102 1 6.9 106.28 . . 95.5 102 2 . . . . 95
102 3 7.5 100.92 73.42 3.399 95 102 4 . 99.08 69.61 3.641 93.2 102 5 4.8 93.67 76.09 3.421 93.1
102 6 . 99.08 . . 94 102 7 6.0 88.27 79.01 0.484 93.2 102 8 . 100.88 . . 93.2
102 9 3.2 102.68 69.75 1.993 94 102 10 . 104.48 . . 94 102 11 8.0 100.88 57.09 0.402 94
102 12 . 99.08 . . . 103 1 8.2 138.71 . . 62 104 1 5.8 178.34 . . 115
105 1 7.7 167.53 . . 110.4 105 2 . . . . 110.3 105 3 3.8 89.37 42.84 3.165 108.1
105 4 . 118.89 42.83 0.614 108.3 105 5 8.1 111.69 63.01 1.530 . 201 1 6.5 122.50 . . 114.1
201 2 . . . . 114.5 201 3 7.8 127.71 33.70 3.176 112.6 201 4 . 127.73 33.64 . 112.3
201 5 7.67 126.10 35.96 3.486 112 201 6 . 124.30 . . 112.3 201 7 6.7 140.51 41.16 3.276 112.3
201 8 . 126.10 . . 112.1 201 9 2.9 131.50 31.72 3.181 113.3 201 10 . 149.52 . . 113
201 11 6.9 136.91 27.12 2.968 112.7 201 12 . 126.10 . . 112.8 201 13 4.0 140.51 . 0.299 112.8
201 14 . 129.70 . . 112.9 201 15 3.2 138.81 71.66 4.059 112.9 201 16 . 156.72 66.54 0.059 113.6
201 17 . 153.12 51.32 0.502 113.2 201 18 . 129.83 41.75 1.197 114 202 1 9.0 194.55 . . 70.9
202 2 . . . . 71.5 202 3 6.3 199.04 78.06 3.333 70.5 202 4 . 167.53 80.32 1.518 71.8
202 5 2.9 156.72 78.35 2.021 70.4 202 6 3.5 217.97 79.29 1.999 70.6
202 7 6.6 163.93 71.61 1.796 71.2 202 8 . 142.31 . . 70.5 202 9 6.0 171.14 79.51 1.422 71
202 10 . 162.13 . . 71 202 11 6.5 160.33 37.18 2.030 70.7 202 12 . 133.30 . . 68.6
202 13 4.2 126.10 72.57 3.553 70 202 14 . 124.30 . . 70 202 15 3.0 143.89 72.91 1.578 70.9
202 16 . 183.75 77.71 3.840 70.9 202 17 . 214.37 77.71 1.055 71
202 18 . 183.54 79.40 0.371 71.5 203 1 12.1 282.83 . . 89.5 204 1 7.1 117.09 . . 116.2
205 1 8.1 147.72 . . 98 205 2 . . . . 98.1 205 3 3.4 125.46 67.81 2.554 98.9
205 4 . 115.29 63.87 3.991 98.5 205 5 3.9 108.08 77.08 1.846 98.3 205 6 . 109.89 . . 99.4
205 7 4.5 120.69 30.86 2.134 97.8 205 8 . 113.49 . . 99.7 205 9 4.9 115.29 44.84 2.440 99.8
205 10 . 113.49 . . 99.4 205 11 6.7 109.89 64.18 3.068 98.7 205 12 . 117.09 . . 99.6
205 13 4.5 120.69 51.78 3.729 98.4 205 14 . 109.89 . . 98.6 205 15 4.8 117.31 73.06 3.934 99.5
205 16 . 129.70 66.60 0.106 97.6 205 17 . 151.32 60.97 0.118 97.2
205 18 . 136.94 48.65 1.632 97.4
;
Run;
```

There's a way to do it better - find it.

---Thomas A. Edison

STEP 5

INTRODUCTION TO PROC STEP

The PROC step consists of a group of SAS statements that call and execute a Procedure. We use PROC Steps to ***analyze*** the data in a SAS data set, produce ***Reports*** or other results. Each PROC has its own unique form with its own list of options. Each Procedure is unique, but there are similarities too. All Procedures have required statements, and most have optional statements.

All Procedures start with the keyword PROC followed by the name of the Procedure, such as PRINT or SORT. Options, if there are any, follow the Procedure name.

Each dataset has two portions 1. Data portion (Data) 2. Descriptor portion (Metadata)

Data Portion:

- ✦ Tabular Arrangement of data
- ✦ Contains Observations and Variables
- ✦ Variables can be either Character or numeric
- ✦ Character variables can be up to 32,767 long
- ✦ Numeric Values stored as floating point variables: have a default length of 8 bytes
- ✦ SAS can handle up to 32,767 variables

Descriptor Portion:

- ✦ Name of the data set
- ✦ Date and time the data set was created
- ✦ Number of observations
- ✦ Number of variables.
- ✦ Variable's attributes like 1.Name, 2.Type, 3.Length, 4.Format, 5.Informat, and 6.Label.

Proc Print (PRINT Procedure)

- The PRINT Procedure produces a display of info from a SAS Dataset. Each observation in the dataset becomes a row on the report, and each variable becomes a column.
- PROC PRINT will use whatever formatting that is already included with the dataset, variables, and other special formatting.
- You can use the ATTRIB, FORMAT, LABEL, and WHERE statements as well as Global statements like TITLE and FOOTNOTE are also used in PROC PRINT.
- You can create a variety of reports ranging from a simple listing to a highly customized report that groups the data and calculates totals and subtotals for numeric variables.

Syntax of PROC Print:

PROC PRINT Options;

BY variable(s);

PAGEBY BY-variable;

SUMBY BY-variable;

ID variable(s);

SUM variable(s);

VAR variable(s);

WHERE Condition;

RUN;

To check the data portion of the dataset and to create simple listing report

PROC Print Data=YLP.Events;

Run;

The ***DATA=*** option is, of course, optional. If you skip it, then SAS will use the most recently created data set in this session i.e. ***_last_.***

- When we execute the above Step, Listing report (***.LST***) will be created in the output window by default.
- In the listing report we observe the Variable Names are reported rather than Variable Labels as in dataset.

- The 'Obs' column is added as the 1st variable and is the number of the observation within the listing.
- The variables are listed in the order in which they were created in the DATA step.

NOOBS option suppresses the display of observation numbers (Obs) in the output (.Lst report).

PROC Print Data=YLP.Events NOOBS;

Run;

LABEL option display variables labels as column headings

Creating a simple listing report with Labels:

PROC Print Data= YLP.Events Obs= 'Observa' Label;

Run;

- In the above code we assigned a column header to Obs variable and created our report with assigned Labels.
- Label specifies a label up to 256 characters.
- Labels are used to replace variable names in SAS output

As per your requirement you can use number of options, but remember that, we tell PROC PRINT what options to use, and it will apply them to the best ability that it can in making the listing report.

VAR statement:

VAR statement - Select variables that appear in the report and ***determine their order***, Otherwise the variables will appear in the order in which they were created.

PROC Print Data= YLP.Events;

VAR Patid Aesev Llterm;

Run;

WHERE Statement:

The WHERE statement enables you to select observations meet one or more conditions.

General form of the WHERE statement:

Where where-expression;

Where-expression is a sequence of operands and operators.

Operands include variables and constants.

Operators include comparison operators, logical operators, special operators and functions.

PROC print data= YLP.Events;

Where aesev = 3;

Run;

Comparison Operators

Mnemonic	symbolic	Definition
EQ	=	equal to
NE	^= ¬= ~=	not equal to
GT	>	greater than
LT	<	Less than
GE	>=	greater than or equal to
IN		equal to one of a list
LE	<=	less than or equal to

Logical Operators

Mnemonic	symbolic	Definition
AND	&	if both expressions are true, then the compound expression is true
OR	|	if either expression is true, then the compound expression is true
NOT	^	can be combined with other operators to reverse the logic of a comparison.

Special Operators

Mnemonic	Symbolic	Definition
BETWEEN-AND		Selects observations in which the value of the variable falls within a range of values, inclusively.
CONTAINS	?	Selects observations that include the specified substring.

To filter the observations based on multiple conditions:

PROC Print Data= YLP.Events;

Where Aesev EQ 2 and Aeout =3;

Run;

While filtering observations based on character variables we need embed the string in quotes, Character comparisons are case-sensitive.

PROC print Data=YLP.Events;

Where Llterm ='dry skin';

Run;

The IN operator allows commas or blanks to separate values.

PROC Print Data= YLP.Events;

Where Aesev in (2, 3);

Run;

***To obtain the data contains the Characters in that sequence*:**

PROC Print Data= YLP.Events;

Where Llterm contains 'hypo';

Run;

IS NULL or IS MISSING selects observations in which the value of the variable is missing.

PROC Print Data = YLP.Events;

Where Aeendt is missing;

Run;

LIKE selects observations by comparing character values to specified patterns.

A percent sign (%) replaces any number of characters.

An underscore (_) replaces one character.

To obtain Llterms starting with d:

PROC Print Data = YLP.Events;

Where Llterm Like 'd%';

Run;

Llterms ends with ia:

PROC Print Data = YLP.Events;

Where Llterm Like '%ia';

Run;

To obtain Llterms contains second letter y:

PROC Print Data = YLP.Events;

Where Llterm Like '_y%';

Run;

Llterms contains t:

PROC Print Data = YLP.Events;

Where Llterm Like '%t%';

Run;

BY Statement

- BY statement - Produce a separate section of the report for each BY group.
- We need to remember that the variable used in by statement should be in ascending order
- To arrange the variable in ascending order we use PROC Sort (Discussed in PROC Sort)
- If the data is not sorted, include the keyword NOTSORTED.

Produce a separate section of the report for each BY group

Proc Print Data=YLP.Vitals;

By Vstest Notsorted;

Run;

PAGEBY Statement

PageBy statement Control page ejects that occurs before a page is full;

PROC Print Data=YLP.Vitals;

By Vstest;

PageBy Vstest;

Run;

SUM Statement

Sum statement gives Total values of numeric variables;

PROC Print Data=YLP.Vitals;

By Vstest;

Sum Vsrn;

Run;

Global Statements:

There are some statements which you can use anywhere in a SAS program these are called global statements.

There are several categories of global statements:

1. Data Access: Libname, Filename Statement
2. Output Control: Title, Footnote Statement
3. Program Control: Options Statement.

Using SAS System Options:

You can use SAS system options to change the appearance of a report.

General form of the OPTIONS statement:

OPTIONS Option…;

The OPTIONS statement is not usually included in a PROC or DATA step.

- ***DATE (default):*** specifies to print the date and time the SAS session began at the top of each page of the SAS output.
- ***NODATE:*** specifies not to print the date and time the SAS session began.
- ***LINESIZE=width, (LS=width):*** specifies the line size for the SAS log and SAS output.
- ***PAGESIZE=n (PS=n):*** specifies the number of lines (n) that can be printed per page of SAS output.
- ***NONUMBER***: specifies that page numbers not be printed.

To suppress the page number

Options nonumber;

By default the PS=56 and LS=120

Options PS=25;

PROC Print Data= YLP.Events;

Run;

To select the observations:

OBS= **system option** specifies an ending point for processing, the FIRSTOBS= system option specifies a starting point. The two options are often used together to define a range of observations to be processed.

Options Firstobs=1 obs=10;

PROC Print Data= YLP.Events;

Run;

The ***OBS= data set option*** specifies an ending point for Processing, the FIRSTOBS= data set option specifies a starting point. The FIRSTOBS= data set option affects a single, existing SAS data set. Use the ***FIRSTOBS=*** system option to affect all steps for the duration of your current SAS session.

*PROC Print Data= YLP.Events (**Firstobs=1 Obs=5**);*

Var Patid Socterm;

Run;

Using Title and Footnote statements:

We use ***Titles*** and ***Footnotes*** to enhance reports.

We can provide up to Ten (10) Titles and Ten (10) Footnotes in a Report

General form of the TITLE statement:

TITLEn 'Text';

Features of Titles and Footnotes:

- Titles appear at the ***top*** of the page while Footnotes appear at the ***bottom*** of the page.
- The value of ***n*** can be from 1 to 10.
- An unnumbered TITLE, FOOTNOTE is equivalent to TITLE1, FOOTNOTE1
- Titles, Footnotes remain in effect until they are changed, cancelled, or you end your SAS session.
- The null TITLE statement, Title; - cancels all titles.

Changing Titles and Footnotes

- TITLEn or FOOTNOTEn replaces a previous title or footnote with the same number and cancels all titles or footnotes with higher numbers.

Title 'Listing 3';

Title2 'Adverse Event Information;

title3 '(Safety Population)';

Footnote 'on 30-Aug-2013';

PROC Print Data= YLP.Events;

Var Patid Aestdt Aeendt;

Run;

Written test question:

Title 'report created by me';

Title2 'On SOC';

Title3 'On Ae dataset';

Title2 'On System Organ Class';

PROC Print Data= YLP.Events (Firstobs=5 Obs=10);

Var Patid Aestdt Aeendt;

Run;

Footnote 'on 30-Aug-2013';

How many titles would be written to the report? What are they?

SAS executes programs line by line the global statements, when executed, latest statement would be in effect that means New Title2 would be replacing the existing Title2 and cancels all the further titles.

Proc Contents (CONTENTS Procedure)

We use Contents Procedure to check the descriptor portion of the dataset. Descriptor portion, even known as Metadata (data about data set), which describes the structure of the data set rather than the data values. PROC Contents displays valuable information at Data set level: (Name, Engine, Creation date, Number of observations, Number of variables, File size (bytes), etc.,) and Variable level: (Name, Type, Length, Formats, Position, Label, etc.,)

PROC Contents Data=YLP.Events;

Run;

By executing the above Procedure we obtained information regarding

1. Attributes
2. Engine/Host info
3. Variables

Attributes (object) info includes dataset name, protection, No. of Obs, No. of Var, Date Created, Date Modified, indexes etc...

Variables attributes includes:

1. *Variable Name*
2. *Type*
3. *Length*
4. *Format*
5. *Informat*
6. *Label*

- ✦ While submitting the project to the Regulatory authorities, we need to submit, the Metadata portion of all the datasets, this metadata is the key submission in the project.

If we want to create a new dataset with descriptor portion details we use OUT= option

PROC Contents Data=YLP.Events Out=Eve_des;

Run;

We are interested in dataset creation, but not the listing report creation. So, we suppress the listing (.Lst) report to save memory, by using NOPRINT option

PROC Contents Data=YLP.Events Out= Eve_des Noprint;

Run;

*Use the **_ALL_** keyword to list all the SAS files in the library and the **NODS** option to suppress the descriptor portions of the data sets. **NODS must be used in conjunction with the keyword _ALL_.***

PROC Contents Data=YLP._ALL_ NODS;

Run;

Print a list of the variables by their position in the data set, use ***VARNUM*** option. The VARNUM option requests the variables to be in the order that they appear in the SAS data set, rather than the default, alphabetical order.

PROC Contents Data=YLP.Events VARNUM;

Run;

Proc Sort (SORT Procedure)

Proc Sort rearranges the order of the observations in a SAS dataset and replaces the dataset, or creates a new dataset.

We use Proc Sort for:

- Rearranges the observations in a SAS data set
- Creates a new SAS data set containing the rearranged observations1
- Sort on one or multiple variables
- Sort in ascending (default) or descending order of by variable
- Do not generate printed output (.lst report)
- treats missing values as the smallest possible value
- We can even perform actions like create a Subset your data, Rename, Drop, Keep, Format, or Label your Variables in the dataset. ;

Rearranges the observations in a SAS data set:

In SAS, Sorts are performed from the leftmost character to the rightmost character of a character variable's value, or on the full numeric value of a numeric variable. Missing numeric values are sorted before any non-missing numeric values.

PROC Sort Data= YLP.Events;

By Aesev;

Run;

By running PROC Sort the original dataset would be modified, To avoid this, we Create a new SAS data set containing the rearranged observations, by using ***OUT=*** Option.

- We use Out= option to create a new output dataset with the result
- The default order is ascending
- When we are arranging the data, missing values takes top position since those values are considered as lowest values

```
PROC Sort Data= YLP.Events Out=Aesrt;
By Patid;
Run;
```

Sometimes it may be useful to ***reverse*** the order of the BY variable. You can do this using the Descending option. This option will sort the data set in descending order by the variable that immediately follows the word ***DESCENDING*** in the BY statement.

```
PROC Sort Data= YLP.Events Out=Des_Ae;
By Descending Aeout;
Run;
```

Sorting on multiple variables:

```
PROC Sort Data= YLP.Events Out=Mulsrt;
By Socterm Pterm;
Run;
```

By executing the above PROC step we sorted the data set, on SOCTERM as first preference, PTERM as second.

Written test question:

```
PROC Sort data= YLP.Events;
By Descending Socterm Pterm;
Run;
```

By executing the above Proc step only Socterm would be arranged in descending order and pterm will be in Ascending order (since we did not specified descending keyword before pterm);

Within the SORT Procedure we can use the DROP=, KEEP= options to Subset Datasets:

```
PROC Sort Data= YLP.Events Out= Aesub (keep=Patid Llterm);
By Patid;
Run;
```

To change the variable name we use Rename option: (Rename= (Old name=New name))

PROC Sort data= YLP.Events Out=Aern (Rename= (Patid=Patient_ID));

By Patid;

Run;

If you use the Rename= option, SAS changes the name of the variable in that Procedure. Second, if you use Rename= with either the Drop= or the Keep= options, the Drop= and the Keep= options are applied before Rename= Thus, use the "old name" in the Drop= and Keep= options. The order in which you place the Rename= Drop= and Keep= options does not matter and does not change Process order.

In regard to using parentheses, a list of multiple variables to rename must be enclosed in parentheses, renaming just one variable does not, and the Keep= variables should not be enclosed in parentheses.

This PROC step works:

PROC Sort data=YLP.Events Out=Aekrn (Rename= (Patid=pt pterm=Aemod) keep=Patid pterm);

By Patid;

Run;

This PROC step yields warning:

PROC Sort Data= YLP.Events Out =Aedrn (Rename= (Patid=Pt Pterm=Aemod) Drop=Pterm);

By Patid;

Run;

WARNING: The variable pterm in the DROP, KEEP, or RENAME list has never been referenced,

Thing to remember is that you cannot Drop and Rename the same variable in the same statement.

Labeling the Variables:

```
PROC Sort Data= YLP.Events Out=Ae_Lbl;
Label Aesev='Adverse Event Severity'
Aerel='Adverse Event Related to Drug';
By Patid;
Run;

PROC Print Data= Ae_Lbl;
Run;
```

By default PROC print creates the .lst report with variable names, if you want to display variable labels, use Label option in PROC print statement

```
PROC Print Data= Ae_Lbl Label;
Run;
```

Using Where= option:

There are times when it is necessary to subset your data, the SORT Procedure allows you to do this by using the WHERE= option or WHERE Statement. Both of these work similarly by selecting observations that meet the condition specified in the WHERE expression before SAS brings them into the PROC SORT for Processing. This may improve the efficiency of your SAS programs because SAS is not required to read all observations from the input dataset.

```
PROC Sort Data=YLP.Events (Where= (Aesev=1)) Out=Aesub;
By Patid;
Run;
```

Using Where statement:

```
PROC sort data= YLP.Events Out=Aesub;
Where Aerel=1;
By Patid;
Run;
```

There may be circumstances when you have a very large data set and you would like to split it up into smaller, more manageable data sets. This may be a time when it would be helpful to use the FIRSTOBS=

and OBS= options within the SORT Procedure. The FIRSTOBS=option causes SAS to begin reading at a specified observation or record. The OBS= option specifies at which observation SAS Processing ends.

PROC Sort Data= YLP.Events (Firstobs=3 obs=5) Out=Aemini;

By Patid;

Run;

The ***NODUPRECS*** (or NODUP) and ***NODUPKEY options*** work similarly in that they both can eliminate unwanted observations, but NODUP compares all the variables in your data set while NODUPKEY compares just the BY variables. More specifically, if you use the ***NODUP option***, PROC SORT compares all variable values for each observation to those for the previous observation that was written to the output data set. If an exact match is found, the observation is not written to the output data set. If you specify the NODUPKEY option, PROC SORT compares all BY variable values for each observation to those for the previous observation written to the output data set. If an exact match using the BY variable values is found, the observation is not written to the output data set.

PROC Sort Data= YLP.Events Out=Aendrs ***NODUP****;*

By Patid;

Run;

PROC sort Data= YLP.Events Nodupkey out=aendk;

By Patid;

Run;

PROC Sort Data= YLP.Events ***Out=*** *unik* ***Dupout****=dup* ***Nodupkey****;*

By Patid;

Run;

By executing the above Proc step, we created two datasets ***unik*** with unique observations based on Patid (by variable) and ***dup*** with repeated observations.

In Clinical Programming we may use Proc Sort to Sort the Events dataset in the following way.

```
PROC sort data= YLP.Events out= unik Nodupkey;
By Patid visid Socterm pterm;
Run;
```

Proc Format (FORMAT Procedure)

A Format is an instruction that SAS uses to write data values.

We use Formats to control the written appearance of data values, or, in some cases, to group data values together for analysis.

Formats are used to change how information is brought into SAS, how it is displayed, and can even be used to reshape the data itself.

The formats in SAS are often used to attach meaning to a coded variable or to change the way data is displayed in the output.

Formats are of two types:

- System defined Formats
- Customized formats

CUSTOMIZED FORMATS

Formats are used to map one value into another. For instance formats are used extensively with SAS dates, which are stored as the number of days since the beginning of time (January 1, 1960).

Since neither you nor your client would like to see the date displayed as 16,014 (November 5, 2003), SAS has provided us with a number of conversion tools that allow us to store the date as a number while displaying it as a text string that we will recognize.

These tools that change how the value is displayed are formats.

There are many formats that SAS has created for handling dates alone. Although there are many formats already created, it is not unusual to have a need to create a specialty format. This can be done with Proc Format and there is a great deal of flexibility as to how the format is created and what it can do for you.

There are two general classes of formats (FORMAT and INFORMAT).Informats are used when reading in data and formats are used to write out values.

Informats and formats can be of three categories:

1. Numeric (w.d), numeric (w.)
2. Character ($w.)
3. Date (w.)

A few selected formats include:

- Dollarw.d includes dollar sign and commas
- Percentw.d writes the number as a percent
- W.d where w is the width and d the number of decimal places
- Zw.d writes leading zeros
- $charw. Writes standard character data preserving leading blanks
- $w. writes standard character data

The application of these formats to the data values on the left could produce the following results:

2345.678 → Dollar9.2 → $2,345.68

0.6723 → Percent8.2 → 67.23%

-0.6723 → Percent8.2 → (67.23%)

2345.678 → 10.2 → 2345.68

2345.678 → Z10.3 → 002345.678

CREATING OUR OWN FORMATS

Although SAS provides a large number of readymade FORMATS and INFORMATS, it is often necessary to create formats designed for a specific purpose.

User defined formats can be used to:

- Convert numeric variables into character values
- Convert character strings into numbers
- Convert character strings into other character strings

The general syntax of the Procedure is:

Proc Format options;

Value Format_name Specifications;

Invalue Informat_name Specifications;

Run;

It is very essential to note that there are some differences between a format name and a variable name:

- A Format name cannot be more than 8 characters
- A Format name cannot end with a number
- A Character format name should always start with the symbol '$'.

The Specifications are made in value pairs.

These pairings are in the form of: Incoming_Value = Formatted_Value;

Advantages of Formats:

- Can be used to manage, analyze and display data
- Enhance visual appeal of reports
- Reduce ambiguity
- Reduce coding
- Centralize Maintenance
- Increase performance
- Creating Formats

```
PROC Format;
Value Genfmt   1= 'Female'
               2= 'Male';
Value Racefmt  1='White'
               2='Black'
               3= 'American Indian';
Run;
```

By executing the above Procedure we created two user defined formats by using ***Value Statement*** and the formats named ***Genfmt*** and ***Racefmt*** (***catalog entries***), which are stored in ***formats catalog*** in ***work library*** by default.

Applying or calling Formats:

Proc Print Data=YLP.Demog;

Format Sex Genfmt. Race Racefmt.;

Run;

Whenever we execute Proc Format the ***Catalog*** named (***formats)*** would be created in ***work library***, with the catalog entries. Since it got created in work library, it is temporary. If we want to make it permanent we need to store the catalog in a permanent library.

Creating a Library to store User Defined Formats:

Libname Fmtlib 'E:\format library';

Creating user defined formats and storing the catalog in Fmtlib:

PROC format Library= Fmtlib;

Value Trtfmt 1='Placebo'

2 = 'Test_Drug 1mg'

3 = 'Test_Drug 3mg'

4 = 'Test_Drug 6mg';

Value Racefmt 1='White'

2='Black'

3= 'American Indian';

Run;

While calling a format, by default SAS searches the formats in WORK library and issues an error message stating that specific format could not be loaded.

Proc Print Data=YLP.Rand;

Format Trtcd Trtfmt.;

Run;

ERROR: The format TRTFMT was not found or could not be loaded.

FORMAT SEARCHES:

Formats are saved in a catalog (usually with the name ***FORMATS***). When requesting a format SAS first checks in WORK.FORMATS and then, if the libref LIBRARY is defined, SAS will look in LIBRARY. FORMATS. Since formats are not usually conveniently located in these two locations, we need to be able to search for formats in a variety of places and in catalogs named something other than FORMATS.

Using FMTSEARCH=:

The FMTSEARCH= system option is used to identify the ***libref*** and ***order for the search***.

Searching the Formats in a specified Library

Options fmtsearch= (Fmtlib);

Once this option is executed, SAS keeps on searching for formats only from that specific library, till the end of the session.

PROC Print Data=YLP.Rand;

Format Trtcd Trtfmt.;

Run;

Once a format is created and saved to a library, we can start to use it in a data step or in a Procedure. If there are multiple format catalogs to be used, it is necessary to specify the format search order by a statement as following.

Options fmtsearch = (Fmtlib Work);

With this option, SAS will search for a format in this order: Fmtlib formats, Work. Formats, if a format cannot be found from all these catalogs, an error message will be issued.

USE A FORMAT LINK AND DE-LINK VARIABLES WITH FORMATS

Sometimes, we may receive a dataset with some variables that have been assigned with permanent formats, but the associated format catalog is not provided. If you still want to use such a dataset, you will need to suppress the Formats xxx was not found" error message by the following OPTIONS statement:

Options nofmterr; (As per SOP, we should not use nofmterr option)

There are other ways to de-link the association between a variable and a format.

```
Data Demog;
Set YLP. Demog;
Format _all_;
Run;
```

This will remove all permanently assigned formats from the data set Demog.

A format statement with only variable names, without any format name, will eliminate any possible format linkage for variables in the list, such as:

```
Data Demog;
Set YLP.Demog;
Format Sex Race;
Run;
```

Any formats, if any, that link with the specified two variables Sex and Race will be removed.

To view the number of catalog entries and their details:

```
PROC Catalog Catalog = FMTLIB. Formats;
Contents;
Run;
Quit;
```

To view the catalog entry values

```
PROC format library = FMTLIB.Formats;
Select Trtfmt Racefmt;
Run;
Quit;
```

If you are changing a format catalog into a data set, you would use the Cntlout = option on the PROC format statement

PROC format Lib = Fmtlib Cntlout =fmtdata;

Select Trtfmt;

Run;

By executing the above step, the Specs of trtfmt in Fmtlib has been sent to a dataset fmtdata.

If you are changing a data set into a format catalog, you would use the Cntlin = option on the PROC format statement.

PROC format Cntlin =fmtdata Lib=YLP;

Run;

By executing the above step, the info in the dataset fmtdata changed as catalog entries in YLP lib

LIST/EXPORT CONTENTS OF A FORMAT:

When we receive a SAS dataset from others, the first thing we need to do is to figure out the contents of the dataset. PROC Contents is a nice tool to do so. For SAS formats, we often need to find out the exact definition of formats too, especially when a set of formats are provided by an outside agency.

If we just need to get a list of formats in a catalog use this:

PROC Catalog Catalog=YLP.Formats;

Contents;

Quit;

The above step will return all the format names, format types and created dates etc in the format catalog. But if we want to get the details of a specific format, we can utilize this code:

PROC Format fmtlib Lib=YLP.Formats;

Select Trtfmt;

Run;

This will list the definitions of the selected format TRTFMT. If we do not specify the SELECT Statement, it will generate the descriptions for all the formats in the catalog.

Creating user defined numeric informats (Invalue Statement):

```
PROC format;
Invalue ginf 'f'=0 'm'=1;
Run;
```

Applying user defined numeric informats

```
Data Test;
Input Id Gen ginf.;
Datalines;
101 m
102 f
103 m
104 M
105 f
;
Run;
```

Written test question:

```
PROC Format;
Value Vfmt 1-50 ='Low'
     51-100='High';
Run;
Data Test;
Input Val @@;
Format Val Vfmt.;
Datalines;
10 15 45 50.5 79 93
;
Run;
```

What would you see in the resultant dataset value 50.5?
a) Low b) High c). d) 50.5

Learning never exhausts the mind.

--Leonardo Da Vinci

STEP 6

COMBINING DATASETS

While creating ADS, Tables, listings and Figures, it is often required to obtain data from more than one dataset, since the required variables might be stored in different datasets, we often Read or Combine data from more than one dataset.

In SAS Clinical Programming, it is almost daily routine for a SAS Clinical Programmer to read Data from two or more SAS Data sets and processing them by:

- Concatenating, Appending
- Interleaving
- One-to-One merging
- match-merging

Concatenating, Appending: Stack Datasets (place one after another).

Interleave: Stack Datasets, but form the result in order by one or more variables present in the Data sets. NOTE: both concatenation and interleaving result in a Dataset that has as many observations as the sum of all the observations in the Data sets being combined.

One-to-One Merge: Combine observation one in Data set one with observation one in Dataset two, observation two-with-two, three-with-three, etc. NOTE: the dataset resulting from one-to-one merge will have as many observations as the number of observations in the largest dataset involved in the merge.

Matched-Merge: Combine observations in datasets based upon the value of one or more variables. NOTE: the number of observations in the resulting dataset depends on the content of the datasets being combined and on the matching options being used.

Concatenating Datasets

Concatenating datasets essentially means stacking one dataset on top of the other, that is, in given two datasets, all of the records from the second dataset will be added to the end of the first dataset.

When concatenating datasets we would expect the datasets to have identical structure but different contents, by structure we mean the tables would have the same columns names and the columns would have the same type (numeric or character).

IF a column exists in one or more of the datasets but not in another, that column is included in all of the Output records but with a missing value for all of the records in the table(s) that did not have that column.

Controlling the Reading and Writing of Variables and Observations:

IF you do not instruct it to do otherwise, SAS writes all variables and all observations from input Datasets to Output Datasets. You can, however, control which variables and observations you want to read and write by using SAS statements, Dataset options, and functions. The statements and Dataset options that you can use are listed in the following table.

Control Variables:

- DROP, KEEP, RENAME --> Statements
- DROP=, KEEP=, RENAME= --> Options

Control Observations:

- WHERE, Subsetting IF --> Statements
- WHERE=, FIRSTOBS=, OBS= --> Options

CONCATENATION

There are a number of methods that can be used to Concatenate Datasets. The easiest, but probably the least efficient way, is to use the ***SET statement.***

```
Data Demo;
Input Patid Site Sex @@;
Datalines;
101 1 2 102 1 1 103 1 1 104 1 1 105 1 1
;
Run;
Data Rand;
Input Patid Trt $ Trtcd @@;
Datalines;
102 6mg 4 105 3mg 3 201 3mg 3 202 3mg 3 205 Placebo 1
;
Run;
Data Test;
Set Demo Rand;
Run;
```

In the resultant dataset Test, we can observe that Since the Patid is common in both the datasets it got appended and Other two variables since they are not matching with first dataset got concatenated.

Appending Datasets

```
Data IC1;
Input Id Site Icdt mmddyy10. @@;
Datalines;
101 1 07-13-2013 103 1 08-26-2013 105 1 09-04-2013
;
Run;
```

```
Data IC2;
Input Id Site Icdt mmddyy10. @@;
Datalines;
102 1 07-28-2010 104 1 08-28-2010
;
Run;
Data Consent;
Set IC1 IC2;
Run;
```

Dataset IC1 is created with three variables: Id, Site, and Icdt. Dataset IC2 is created with the same three variables: Id, Site, and Icdt. The two Datasets are combined with a SET statement. The Output dataset shows the two data sets combined Top-to-bottom.

You can concatenate as many Datasets as you want with a SET statement. This method forces SAS to read every observation in each of the Datasets being combined. Concatenation using the SET statement is very robust, i.e. there are not many conditions that will cause it to fail.

However, concatenation using SET is sensitive to the ***Type of variables*** in the datasets. You cannot have a variable with the same name across datasets defined as Numeric in one dataset and as Character in another. IF Id Variable had been Numeric in DATA set IC1 and Character in Dataset IC2, the Datasets could not be combined and the following error would appear in the LOG when the Datasets were used in the same SET statement.

ERROR: Variable ID has been defined as both character and numeric.

```
Data IC1;
Input Id Country $3. +1 Icdt ddmmyy10.;
Datalines;
101 Ind 20-03-2010
103 Ind 20-03-2010
105 Ind 20-03-2010
;
Run;
```

```
Data IC2;
Input Id Site Country $ Icdt ddmmyy10.;
Datalines;
102 1 India 24-03-2010
104 1 India 24-03-2010
106 1 India 24-03-2010
108 1 India 24-03-2010
;
Run;

Data Apen;
Set IC1 IC2;
Run;
```

Dataset IC1 is created with three variables: Id Country Icdt Country has a length of 3. Dataset IC2 is created with four variables: Id Site Country Icdt and Country has a length of 8. The Datasets are combined using SET Statement.

The variable Country had a length of 3 in Dataset IC1, since Dataset IC1 occurs first in the SET statement, the length of variable Country in the combined Dataset is also 3 and the names from Dataset IC2 are truncated. A LENGTH statement in the Data step that combines IC1 and IC2 would override this problem, or just change the order of the Datasets in the SET statement.

PROC APPEND (Append Procedure):

Proc Append is a more efficient way to concatenate Datasets than SET. However, only two Datasets can be combined at one time, a BASE dataset and a DATA dataset. Observations from the DATA dataset are added to the end of the BASE dataset.

Concatenation via Proc Append is less robust than concatenation via SET. Proc Append is sensitive not only to the TYPE of variables in the two DATA sets, but also to what variables are present in each DATA set, and their lengths.

Proc Append BASE=IC1 DATA=IC2;

Run;

WARNING: Variable site was not found on BASE file.

WARNING: Variable Country has different lengths on BASE and DATA

ERROR: No appending done because of anomalies listed above. Use FORCE option to append these files.

NOTE: 0 observations added.

NOTE: The DATA set WORK.IC1 has 3 observations and 3 variables.

NOTE: Statements not processed because of errors noted above.

Due to the differences noted in the LOG, Proc Append will not combine the DATA sets. IF you want to override these limitations, you can use the FORCE option (but be careful).

Proc append base=IC1 DATA=IC2 ***FORCE****;*

Run;

The FORCE option is used with PROC APPEND.

There are warnings but no errors in the log file. The Datasets are combined.

The variable site is not in the combined Dataset.

The variable Country has the same length as Country in the base Dataset IC1.

The combined Dataset ends up with the same name as the BASE Dataset.

Unlike combining Datasets with a SET statement, variables in the Dataset not present in the BASE dataset are dropped from the combined Dataset.

The lengths of variables are controlled by those in the BASE Dataset.

With all these additional limitations, Proc Append might seem less useful than combining Datasets with a SET statement. The advantage of Proc Append is EFFICIENCY.

Interleaving Datasets

Interleaving is ***'Sorted Concatenation'*** and is done using a SET statement and a BY variable(s). When a BY statement is used with a SET statement that specifies two or more datasets, the DATA step reads the two or more files simultaneously, alternating sequentially between the files based on the lowest level groupings of the BY variables. This has the advantage of maintaining the sort order of the Data from the datasets as they are jointly processed.

For example, suppose there are two datasets, one for males and one for females, and both are sorted on Age. They can be interleaved into a single dataset sorted on Age and Gender. Since the values of Sex are unique within each dataset, the variable may be included on the BY statement even though it is not explicitly sorted.

```
Proc Sort Data=YLP.Demog Out=Male;
By Birthyr;
Where Sex=2;
Run;

Proc Sort Data=YLP.Demog Out=Female;
By Birthyr;
Where Sex=1;
Run;

Data Demog;
Set Male Female;
By Birthyr Sex;
Run;
Proc sort Data=IC1;
By Id;
Run;
```

```
DATA IC2mod;
Input Id Site Country $3. +1 Icdt ddmmyy10.;
Datalines;
102 1 Ind 24-03-2010
104 1 Ind 24-03-2010
106 1 Ind 24-03-2010
108 1 Ind 24-03-2010
;
Run;
Proc sort DATA=IC2mod;
By Id;
Run;
Data Ic_Intlv;
Set IC1 IC2mod;
By Id;
Run;
```

Both Datasets are sorted by variable Id. The Datasets are combined with a SET statement, plus a BY statement. IF the combined Dataset is very large, it may be more efficient to first sort the smaller Datasets THEN use SET and BY to interleave.

Merging Datasets

The MERGE statement joins corresponding observations from two or more SAS Datasets into single observations in a new SAS Dataset.

The way the SAS system joins the observations depends on whether a BY statement accompanies the MERGE statement or not there are different types of merges

- One-to-One,
- One-to-Many, Many-to-One,
- Many-to-Many.

ONE-TO-ONE MERGE:

Concatenation and interleaving combine datasets ***'top-to-bottom'*** - observations in one dataset are added to observations in another dataset. Merging combines datasets ***'side-to-side'*** - variables in one dataset are added to variables in another dataset.

One-to-One merge combine observation #1 in dataset one with observation #1 in dataset two, #2 with #2, and so on.

SAS checks the dataset mentioned on the right. IF you have variables with the same names in datasets that are being merged, SAS will keep the values of the variables from the right-most named dataset in the ***MERGE statement***.

A one-to-one merge is only useful when you are sure that the order of the observations in the Datasets being combined is appropriate, i.e. observation #1 in Dataset one should be combined with #1 in Dataset two.

Default Merge: One to one, No Matching

Each observation from dataset one is combined with a corresponding observation in dataset two. The default action taken by SAS when the code requests a merger between two datasets is to simply combine the observations one by one in the order that they appear in the datasets.

Positional merge with common variable and without specifying by statement;

```
DATA Demo;
Input Id Gender $ @@;
Datalines;
101 male 103 female 104 female
;
Run;
DATA Preg;
Input Id Preg_YN $;
Datalines;
103 Yes 104 Yes 106 No
;
Run;
```

```
DATA Posi_mer;
Merge Demo Preg;
Run;
```

Executing the above step, the Id variable in second dataset over writes on Id variable of first dataset and gives unexpected result.

One to one Merge with by statement

```
DATA Cor_Mer;
Merge Demo Preg;
By Id;
Run;
```

MATCHED MERGE:

Matched merging is Side-to-Side combination of datasets in which observations are combined on the basis of the value(s) of one or more variables, i.e. BY variable(s). Since a By-variable is used, all Datasets in the MERGE statement must be sorted in order of that by variable.

```
Data DOB;
Input Id Gen $ Birthdt ddmmyy10. @@;
Datalines;
101 m 20-03-1975 103 f 25-08-1965 104 m 12-03-1954 105 m 12-12-1980
;
Run;

DATA ICD;
Input Id Icdt ddmmyy10. @@;
Datalines;
101 23-03-2010 102 25-03-2010 105 20-03-2010
;
Run;
```

Here, both DOB and ICD are in sorted order on ID variable so no sorts are done. Dataset Combine is now 'correct' in that it contains matched records, plus the extra unmatched observations.

```
Data Combine;
Merge DOB ICD;
By id;
Run;
```

In a merge, common variables that are not part of BY statement, act as follows: the values coming in from the right dataset override those coming in from the left dataset.

```
Data DOB;
Input Id Date ddmmyy10. @@;
Datalines;
101 20-03-1975 103 25-08-1965 105 12-03-1954
;
Run;

Data ICD;
Input Id Date ddmmyy10. @@;
Datalines;
101 23-03-2010 103 25-03-2010 104 20-03-2010 107 21-03-2010
;
Run;

Data Combine;
Merge DOB ICD;
By Id;
Run;
```

By executing the above step the date variable from ICD dataset override on date variable on DOB dataset, But SAS does not issue any message in the log window.

To raise this issue in the log window we use Msglevel=I option (By default Msglevel=N);

```
Options Msglevel=I;
DATA Combine;
Merge DOB ICD;
By Id;
Run;
```

By using Msglevel=I option we get the INFO: in the log window stating that the variable date on dataset work.dob will be overwritten by dataset work.icd.

INFO: The variable Date on data set WORK.DOB will be overwritten by data set WORK.ICD.

The work around for this problem is to rename date variable in any dataset; Renaming the variable

```
DATA IC;
Set ICD;
Rename Date= Icdt;
Run;

Options Msglevel=I;
DATA Combine;
Merge DOB IC;
By Id;
Run;
```

MATCH MERGE

- In the match-merge, there were instances when observations in one DATA set did not match any observations in the other DATA set.
- IF we want to keep paired observations in the DATA set that results from a merge, i.e. observations with contributions from both DATA sets.

```
Data Events;
Input id Ae $;
Datalines;
101 Headache 104 Vomit 107 Anorexia 108 Bodypain 109 Bodypain
;
Run;

Data Conmed;
Input id cm $;
Datalines;
101 Nise 103 Crocin 104 Vomistop 105 Nise 108 Anacin
;
Run;

To obtain common obs on by variable
Data aecm;
Merge Events (In=inae) Conmed (In=incm);
By id;
IF inae and incm;
Run;
```

- ✦ A new option is added to both Datasets in the merge statement, i.e., IN=.
- ✦ Two new variables are created with the ***IN= option***, Inae and Incm.
- ✦ Variables Inae and Incm are checked. IF an observation contributes variables to a matched observation, the value of a variable created with IN= will be 1, otherwise it will have a value of 0.
- ✦ Dataset AECM has only matched observations.
- ✦ An IN option is used on each Dataset involved in the merge.

- The IN option variables, in this case Inae and Incm, can be assigned any valid SAS names and these variables only exist for the duration of the DATA step and they will not appear in Dataset AECM. The values of Inae and Incm are contingent upon whether the Dataset with which they are associated contributes variables to an observation formed by the MERGE statement.

IF we want to keep all observations from AE whether or not they are matched to an observation in CM, we can rewrite the DATA step as.

```
DATA Aeonly;
Merge Events (IN=Inae) Conmed (IN=Incm);
By id;
IF Inae;
Run;
```

- The only IN= variable added to the DATA step is associated with dataset AE. The Subsetting IF statement only checks to see IF an observation contains information from an observation in the AE dataset.
- The IN= variable(s) can also be used to create multiple datasets during a DATA step merge.
- What IF all the matched observations were to be put in one DATA set, observations from Ae dataset in another, and unmatched observations put in another.

```
Data aecm onlyae onlycm;
Merge Events (in=inae) Conmed (in=incm);
By id;
IF not incm THEN Output onlyae;
IF inae and incm THEN Output aecm;
IF not inae THEN Output onlycm;
Run;
```

Performing One - Many Merge:

IF there are multiple observations with the same value of the by variable in one of the datasets being merged, the term one-to-many match merge (or many-to-one match merge) is used.

```
Data rand;
Input id trt $ @@;
Datalines;
101 Active 102 Placebo 103 Active 104 Active
;
Run;
Data Events;
Length id 4 aeterm $ 12;
Input id aeterm $ @@;
Datalines;
101 Vomit 101 Headache 103 Nausea 104 Insomnia 104 Anorexia 104 Palpitations
;
Run;
Data Combine;
Merge Rand Events;
By Id;
Run;
```

Performing Many - One Merge:

```
Data Demog;
Input Pat_Ini $ age @@;
Datalines;
ALR 20 KKR 21 VSR 50 VSR 33
;
Run;
```

```
Data Vitals;
Input Pat_Ini $ HR @@;
Label hr = 'heart rate';
Datalines;
ALR 89 KKR 98 VSR 91
;
Run;

Data both;
Merge Demog vitals;
By Pat_Ini;
Run;
```

- The first Dataset contains demographic data.
- The second Dataset contains Vitals data.
- Demographic and Vitals data are combined using merge with a By variable.
- Each VSR (Many) in Dataset demographic was combined with VSR (One) in Dataset Vitals.
- In a matched merge, the BY statement causes SAS to look for possible matches based on the value of the by-variable(s).

You renew yourself every day. Sometimes you're successful, sometimes you're not, but it's the average that counts.

--Satya Nadella

STEP 7

SAS FUNCTIONS

INTRODUCTION

In our day to day clinical programming tasks, we need to modify, manipulate, and transform data in order to make the data ready for Analysis and Reporting. We use some or other ***Function*** for most data manipulations. Familiarity with these functions can make programming much easier.

A FUNCTION is a built-in method and returns a value from a computation or system manipulation that requires zero or more arguments.

The SAS System provides an extensive library of built-in functions

Syntax of function

New_Var = Funtion_Name (Req_argument1 .., Opt_argument1 ....N);

Features of SAS functions:

- A function recognized in a SAS statement by the use of a function name, followed immediately by function argument(s), separated by commas, and enclosed in parentheses
- However, the number of required and optional arguments varies (Zero to Many).
- Some functions simply have one required argument.
- Others have one required and one or more optional arguments.
- Functions that are more complex may have several required arguments.
- In most cases, the order of the arguments is important.
- Some people may think that if the code runs, then they had the arguments in the right order but that isn't always the case.

- Some functions will give different results if you accidentally swap the order of the arguments.
- Some functions take no arguments, in which case a Null set of parentheses is required

The arguments to any given function can be

- Variables---Y = ABS(Var_Name) ;
- Constants---X = SQRT(9562) ;
- Expressions---- Z = MAX(Pre-Post) ;
- Functions ---Q = Left(Trim(Str));

Arithmetic Functions

ABS Function: We use this function to obtain the ***Absolute Value*** (Negative values to positive).

```
Data _NULL_;
FILE 'E:\nulrpt.txt';
Val= -17;
Abs_Val = ABS (Val);
PUT Abs_Val =;
Run;
```

In clinical studies, Patient visits are scheduled in Protocol. Let us assume in study X, Visits are planned on Day1, Day30, Day60, Day120 for Visit3, Visit4, Visit5, Visit6 respectively (As per Protocol). Patients are allowed to have 3 day Window period.

```
Data Window;
Input Patid Visnum Plan_day Act_day Vsrn @@;
Datalines;
1001 3 1 1 78 1001 3 1 2 82 1001 4 30 29 83 1001 4 30 30 88 1001 4 30 31 82
1001 5 60 56 79 1001 5 60 63 80 1001 6 120 115 67 1001 6 120 125 77
;
Run;
```

Data Win_Mod;

Set Window;

Diff= ABS (Plan_day - Act_day);

Run;

DATA _NULL_: The ***Data set name _NULL_*** is a special keyword. The _NULL_ Data set does not get saved into workspace. The keyword turns off all the default automatic output that normally occurs at the end of the Data step. It is used typically for writing output to reports or files.

FILE statement: Routes the output from the PUT statement to either the same external file to which procedure output is written or to a different external file.

PUT statement: Writes lines to the SAS log, the output file, or any file that is specified in a FILE statement. If no FILE statement has been executed in this iteration of the DATA step, then the PUT statement writes, to the SAS log.

MOD Function: Returns the remainder from the division of the first argument by the second argument, fuzzed to avoid most unexpected floating-point results.

Syntax: *New_Var=MOD (Argument1, Argument2);*

- Argument-1: is a numeric constant, variable, or expression that specifies the dividend.
- Argument-2: is a numeric constant, variable, or expression that specifies the divisor.

Data Test;

Val= MOD (22, 4);

Run;

By executing the above step we created a dataset named Test with a variable VAL, The data value of this variable is 2 which is the remainder from the division.

Character Functions

UPCASE, LOWCASE AND PROPCASE FUNCTIONS:

In Clinical studies we may receive data from different sites and each site may enter data in their preferred way (Upper, Lower Case). When we need to work on such data, we may want to convert all of our character values in one case, UPCASE, PROPCASE, or LOWCASE.

Remember that upper and lowercase values are represented by different internal codes, so if you are testing for a value such as **R** for a variable and the actual value is **r**, you will not get a match. Therefore it is often useful to convert all character values to either upper- or lowercase before doing your logical comparisons.

- These three functions change the case of the argument.
- UPCASE and LOWCASE change the case of characters to Upper, Lower respectively.
- PROPCASE (stands for proper case) capitalizes the first character in each 'word' and sets the remaining letters to lowercase.
- The default delimiter is a space so the PROPCASE function will capitalize each word.
- You can specify a list of delimiters as the optional second argument to this function.

Here is an example

```
Data _Null_;
SOCTERM='Cardiac disorders';
Up_Soc= Upcase (SOCTERM);
Lo_Soc = Lowcase (SOCTERM);
Prop_Soc = Propcase (SOCTERM);
Put Up_Soc = Lo_Soc = Prop_Soc =;
Run;
```

If we get the Data like this, the task is to create a new dataset contains the subjects who randomized to Active Treatment and got Adverse Events

```
Data Test;
Length Patid 3 Trt $7 AE $10;
Input Patid Trt $  AE $;
Datalines;
101 active nausea
102 placebo no
105 active No
108 Active insomnia
109 ACTIVE Dizziness
110 Placebo Bodypain
;
Run;
```

Converting the cases of both TRT and AE to uppercase

```
Data Modi;
Set Test;
Trtup = Upcase (Trt);
Aeup = Upcase (Ae);
Run;

Data Final (Drop=Trtup Aeup);
Set Modi;
Where Trtup='ACTIVE' and Aeup ne 'NO';
Run;
```

ANY FUNCTIONS:

These functions return the first position of ANY DIGIT, ALPHA, ALNUM, PUNCT or SPACE in the String of characters.

Syntax: ANY** (String, Startpos);***

- DIGIT = any digit
- ALPHA = any character

- ALNUM = any character or digit
- PUNCT = any punctuation
- SPACE = any space

ANYALNUM FUNCTION: We use this function to locate the first occurrence of an alphanumeric character (any upper- or lowercase letter or number) and return its position. If none is found, the function returns a 0. With the use of an optional parameter, this function can begin searching at any position in the String and can also search from right to left, if desired.

Syntax: *ANYALNUM (character-value <, start>);*

If the start value is positive, the search goes from left to right; if the value is negative, the search goes from right to left.

```
Data _Null_;
String = 'S02-P107 has Nausea';
ADF1= ANYDIGIT (String);
ADF2= ANYDIGIT (String,6);
ADF3= ANYDIGIT (String,-25);
APF= ANYPUNCT (String);
ASF=ANYSPACE (String);
AAF=ANYALPHA (String);
AANF=ANYALNUM (String);
Put ADF1= ADF2= ADF3= APF= ASF= AAF= AANF=;
Run;
```

- ANYDIGIT (String): searches for any digit and returns the position of 2 which is for number '1';
- ANYDIGIT (String, 6) searches for any digit in the String starting from position 6 and returns the position of 8 which is for number '1'. ;
- ANYDIGIT (String,-25) searches for any digit in the String starting from -25 or backward and returns the position of 10 which is for number '8'. Note: the search is backward but position returned is relative to the starting position.
- ANYPUNCT (String) searches for any punctuation in the String and returns the position of 4 which is for '-'

- ANYSPACE (String) searches for any punctuation in the String and returns the position of 9 which is for ' '
- ANYALPHA (String) searches for any character in the String and returns the position of 1 which is for character 'S'.
- ANYALNUM (String) searches for any character or digit in the String and returns the position of 1 which is for character 'S'.

INDEX, INDEXC AND INDEXW FUNCTIONS

INDEX and INDEXC functions return the position where the char or String of characters first occurs in the String. INDEXW function searches for entire word.

Syntax:

- INDEX (String, Search String)
- INDEXC (String, Search String)
- INDEXW (String, Search Word)

```
Data _Null_;
String = 'THIS IS SASI, A SAS ANALYST';
Ind_val = INDEX (String, 'SAS');
Indc_val = INDEXC (String, 'SAS');
Indw_val = INDEXW (String, 'SAS');
Put Ind_val = Indc_val = Indw_val =;
Run;
```

INDEX (String, 'SAS') searches for the substring 'SAS' in the String and returns the position of Nine (9) when it encounters the String SAS i.e., in SASI.

INDEXC (String, 'SAS') searches the String for either 'S' or 'A' and returns the position of Four (4) which is when it first encounters letter 'S'. i.e., in THIS

INDEXW (String, 'SAS') searches the String for the word 'SAS' and returns the position of 17 where if first finds 'SAS' i.e., exact word SAS.

FIND, FINDC AND FINDW FUNCTIONS

The purpose of FIND function is to locate a substring within a String. With optional arguments, you can define the starting point for the search, the direction of the search, and ignore case or trailing blanks. FINDC function is to locate a character that appears or does not appear within a String. With optional arguments, you can define the starting point for the search, the direction of the search, to ignore case or trailing blanks, or to look for characters except the ones listed

Syntax:

- FIND (String, Search String, Startpos, Modifier);
- FINDC (String, Search String, Startpos, Modifier);

The find function also searches for a Search string in a string, but allows "***modifiers***" and a "***starting position***" to be specified. Two modifiers exist, "i" and "t". The "i" modifier tells SAS to ***ignore*** the Case, the "t" modifier ***trims*** trailing blanks from the String. The starting position tells SAS from which position in the string ***to start***.

```
Data _Null_;
String='This is SASI, a SAS Analyst';
Fnd_Val = Find (String, 'S');
Fndi_Val =Find (String, 'S', 'i');
Fndsp_val =Find (String, 'S',15);
Put Fnd_Val= Fndi_Val= Fndsp_val=;
Run;
```

COUNT and COUNTC Functions:

These functions count the occurrences of a String in a bigger character String. ;

Syntax:

- COUNT (String, Search String, <Modifier>);
- COUNTC (String, Search String, <Modifier>);

Modifiers: I = Ignore Case, T = Remove Leading and Trailing Blanks

```
Data _Null_;
String = 'Lp lp de lp LP gh lp';
Nst_Val = COUNT (String, 'lp');
Cst_Val = COUNT (String, 'LP');
Ict_Val = COUNT (String, 'lp', 'I');
Ccnt_Val = COUNTC (String, 'lp');
Iccnt_Val = COUNTC (String, 'lp', 'I');
Put Nst_Val = Cst_Val = Ict_Val = Ccnt_Val = Iccnt_Val =;
Run;
```

- Nst_Val count all the occurrences of 'lp' in the String and hence returns a value of 3.
- Cst_Val count all the occurrences of 'LP' in the String and returns a value of 1.
- Ict_Val count all the occurrences of 'lp' and 'LP' due to 'I' modifier in the String and hence returns value of 5.
- Ccnt_Val count all the occurrences of 'l' as well as 'p' in the String and hence return the value of 7.
- Iccnt_Val count all the occurrences of 'l','L','p' and 'P' in the String due to the 'I' modifier and hence returns the value of 10.

LEFT, RIGHT Functions:

These functions left or right align text. Remember that the length of a character variable will not change when you use these two functions. If there are leading blanks, the LEFT function will shift the first non-blank character to the first position and move the extra blanks to the end; if there are trailing blanks, the RIGHT function will shift the non-blank text to the right and move the extra blanks to the left.

LEFT Function: To left-align text values, LEFT doesn't "remove" the leading blanks; it moves them to the end of the String. Thus, it doesn't change the storage length of the variable, even when you assign the result of LEFT to a new variable. The LEFT function is particularly useful if values were read with the $CHAR informat, which preserves leading blanks.

Syntax: *LEFT (character-value)*

RIGHT Function: To right-align a text String. Note that if the length of a character variable has previously been defined and it contains trailing blanks, the RIGHT function will move the characters to the end of the String and add the blanks to the beginning so that the final length of the variable remains the same.

Syntax: RIGHT (character-value)

Trimming and Concatenation Functions:

Very often, the DATA you receive might contain unwanted spaces, and you want to remove them to make your DATA clean. SAS provides a variety of useful character functions to handle blanks in a character String.

Some frequently used functions that remove leading blanks, trailing blanks or multiple blanks in the middle of a String. The purpose is to make DATA manipulation more accurate, efficient. The functions include TRIM, TRIMN, STRIP, LEFT, COMPRESS, COMPBL, and a few concatenation functions including CAT, CATT, CATS, and CATX.

TRIM, TRIMN, and STRIP Functions:

The two functions TRIM and TRIMN are similar: they both remove trailing blanks from a String. The functions work identically except when the argument contains only blanks. In that case, TRIM returns a single blank (length of 1) and TRIMN returns a Null String with a length of 0. The STRIP function removes both leading and trailing blanks.

TRIM Function: To remove trailing blanks from a character value. This is especially useful when you want to concatenate several Strings together and each String may contain trailing blanks. Important note: The length of the variable returned by the TRIM function will be the same length as the argument, unless the length of this variable has been previously defined.

Syntax: TRIM (character-value)

```
Data Test;
Length T_FullName $ 30;
Informat NAME1 NAME2 $15.;
Infile Datalines Missover;
Input NAME1 NAME2 NAME3;
T_FullName = TRIM (NAME1) || ' ' || TRIM (NAME2);
FullName = NAME1 || NAME2;
Keep T_FullName FullName;
Datalines;
Sriram Prakhyath
 David Anand
Mahesh Iyer
;
Run;
```

To put the names together, you use the concatenate operator (||). The TRIM function is used to trim trailing blanks from each of the words (which are all 15 bytes in length), before putting them together. Without the TRIM function, there are extra spaces between each of the names

STRIP Function:

- To strip leading, trailing blanks from character variables or Strings.
- STRIP (CHAR) is equivalent to TRIMN (LEFT(CHAR)), but more convenient.

Syntax: STRIP (character-value)

Character-value is any SAS character expression. If the STRIP function is used to create a new variable, the length of that new variable will be equal to the length of the argument of the STRIP function. If leading or trailing blanks were trimmed, trailing blanks will be added to the result to pad out the length as necessary. The STRIP function is useful when using the concatenation operator.

```
Data _NULL_;
ONE = "   S101   "; *Note: three leading and trailing blanks;
TWO = "   P107   "; *Note: three leading and trailing blanks;
N_STP = ":" || ONE || "-" || TWO || ":";
STP = ":" || STRIP(ONE) || "-" || STRIP(TWO) || ":";
PUT ONE= TWO= / N_STP= / STP=;
RUN;
```

Functions That Join Two or More Strings Together:

Although you can use the || concatenation operator in combination with the STRIP, TRIM, or LEFT functions, concatenation functions make it much easier to put Strings together and, if you wish, to place one or more separator characters between the Strings.

CAT Functions (CAT, CATS, CATT, and CATX):

CAT Function is to concatenate (join) two or more character Strings, leaving leading and/or trailing blanks unchanged. This function accomplishes the same task as the concatenation operator (||).

Syntax: CAT (String-1, String-2 <, String-n>)

CATT Function is to concatenate (join) two or more character Strings, stripping only trailing blanks.

Syntax: CATT (String-1, String-2 <, String-n>)

CATS Function is to concatenate (join) two or more character Strings, stripping both leading and trailing blanks.

Syntax: CATS (String-1, String-2 <, String-n>)

CATX Function is to concatenate (join) two or more character Strings, stripping both leading and trailing blanks and inserting one or more separator characters between the Strings.

Syntax: CATX (Separator, String-1, String-2 <, String-n>)

Separator is one or more characters, placed in single or double quotation marks, to be used as separators between the concatenated Strings.

Note: It is very important to set the length of the resulting character String, using a LENGTH statement (or other method), before using any of the concatenation functions. Otherwise, the length of the resulting String will default to 200.

```
Data CAT_Test;
String1 = "LAB"; * No spaces;
String2 = "Test   "; * Three trailing spaces;
String3 = "   ^"; * Three leading spaces;
String4 = "   Test   "; * Three leading and trailing spaces;
LENGTH Result1 – Result4 $ 20;
Result1 = CAT (String1, String3);
Result2 = CATS (String1, String4);
Result3 = CATT (String2, String1);
Result4 = CATX (", ", String1, String4);
RUN;

PROC PRINT DATA=CAT_Test NOOBS;
RUN;
```

Notice that each of the STRING variables differs with respect to leading and trailing blanks.

The CAT function is identical to the || operator. The CATS function removes both leading and trailing blanks and is equivalent to TRIM (LEFT (STRING2)) || TRIM (LEFT (STRING4). The CATT function, trims only trailing blanks. The last statements use the CATX function, which removes leading and trailing blanks. It is just like the CATS function but adds one or more separator characters (specified as the first argument), between each of the Strings to be joined.

COMPRESS Function

Compress function Compresses/removes blanks (By default) or specified characters from a given String.

Syntax: New_Var = Compress (String,,);

```
Data _Null_;
String = ' Y     Lakshmi     Prasad ';
Cmp_Str = COMPRESS (String);
Put String =;
Put Cmp_Str =;
Run;
```

COMPRESS Function with the second Argument:

Data _Null_;

Mob_Num='n897-878-+ +/&4848';

Cmp_Num = COMPRESS (Mob_Num, 'n -');

Put Mob_Num =;

Put Cmp_Num =;

Run;

COMPRESS Function with the Third Argument:

Modifiers that can be used are:

K = Keep

I = Ignore case

D = Digits

A = Alpha (upper and lower)

S = Space

P = Punctuations

Data Test;

String= 'Sasi 905-911-9070';

Cmp_V1= COMPRESS (String, 'S', 'I');

Cmp_V2= COMPRESS (String, , 'A');

Cmp_V3= COMPRESS (String, , 'P');

Cmp_V4= COMPRESS (String, , 'KDS');

Cmp_V5= COMPRESS (String, '0', 'KDS');

Run;

Cmp_V1: Compress (String, 'S', 'I') would compress the letter 'S' and with the modifier 'I' case would be ignored .So this will compress 'S' and 's'.

Cmp_V2: Compress(String, , 'A') does not have the second argument but has the modifier 'a' which says drop Alpha (upper and Lower).Hence all the alphabets from the String are compressed.

Cmp_V3: Compress (String, , 'P') does not have the second argument but has the modifier 'p' which says drop punctuations. Hence all the punctuations from the String are compressed. Note that the blank spaces are not part of punctuations and hence are not compressed.

Cmp_V4: Compress(String, , 'KDS') does not have the second argument but has the modifiers 'KDS' which say 'Keep', 'Digits' and 'Space'. Hence only digits and spaces from the String are kept.

Cmp_V5: Compress (String,'0', 'KDS') has a second argument and also additional modifiers. Second argument '0' instructs to compress all Zero's in the String. However the third argument 'KDS' instructs to keep all digits and space. As observed in the output the third argument takes precedence over the second argument.

The COMPRESS function with the third argument (new modifiers) can be very handy to simplify our code and reduce chances of errors.

COMPBL Function:

Compress Blank or Compbl function is used to convert multiple blanks to a single blank. It is really useful when we have a long String of words which may be separated by multiple blanks and we need to convert those to a single blank. COMPRESS function can remove not only blanks, but also any characters you specify from a String.

Syntax: New_Var = COMPBL (String);

```
Data Test;
Aeterm='Dry      Skin';
Ae_cbl = Compbl (Aeterm);
Run;
```

REPEAT Function: Repeat Function is to make multiple copies of a String.

Syntax: REPEAT (character-value, n)

- Character-value is any SAS character expression.
- n is the number of repetitions.

The result of this function is the original String plus n repetitions. Thus if n equals 1, the result will be two copies of the original String in the result. If you do not declare the length of the character variable holding the result of the REPEAT function, it will default to 200.

Functions That Compute the Length of Strings:

LENGTH function: To determine the length of a character value, not counting trailing blanks. A Null argument returns a value of 1.

Syntax: LENGTH (character-value)

- The LENGTH and LENGTHN functions return the length of a character variable, not counting trailing blanks.
- The only difference between the LENGTH and LENGTHN functions is that the LENGTH function returns a value of 1 for a Null String while the LENGTHN function returns a 0.
- The LENGTHC function does count trailing blanks in its calculations. Finally, the LENGTHM function returns the number of bytes of memory used to store the variable.

Data Test;

*String1= '   Nausea   '; *String with three leading and three trailing blanks;*

*String2= ' '; *Empty String;*

len_str1= length (String1);

lenn_str1= lengthn (String1);

lenc_str1 = lengthc (String1);

len_estr2 = length (String2);

lenn_esst2 = lengthn (String2);

Run;

PUT and INPUT Functions: PUT and INPUT are useful for converting variables from character to numeric and the reverse.

PUT Function Converts from a numeric or character variable/target to a character output, applying a format as part of the conversion. The Put function can be applied to a character or numeric input, but the output of the Put function is always character.

INPUT Function Converts only from a character variable/target to either numeric or character output/variables, applying an Informat as part of the conversion. The INPUT Function can only be applied to a character target, but the output can be character or numeric.

CONVERTING NUMERIC VARIABLES TO CHARECTER VARIABLES

The simplest way to convert numeric data to character data is using the PUT function. Converting numbers to characters is quite easy. If you have only whole numbers use the following statement:

Char_var = PUT (Num_var, 8.);

If you have numeric data (subject numbers for example). If you want to convert to a character variable and still have the sort sequentially then you must zero fill the data.

Char_var = STRIP (PUT (Num_var, z2.));

```
Data Test;
Input Patid @@;
Datalines;
1 5 9 13 17 21
;
Run;

Data Test_fun;
Set Test;
Sub_C= PUT (Patid, 2.);
Subj_Lz = STRIP (PUT (Patid, z2.));
Run;
```

> If you want to add trailing zeroes to the data you use the following:
> Char_var = STRIP (PUT (Num_var, 8.2)); This will store the data out to 2 decimal places

```
Data Test;
Input Lbrn @@;
Datalines;
11.65 12.2 10.345 10.6574
;
Run;
```

Data Test_fun;

Set test;

LB_RC =PUT (Lbrn, 7.4);

Run;

CONVERTING CHARACTER VARIABLES TO NUMERIC VARIABLES

The simplest way to convert Character data to Numeric data is using the INPUT function. If you have only numeric data as an integer in a character variable use the following statement:

Num_var = INPUT (Char_var, 8.);

Because a numeric variable does not display trailing zeroes in the output. The easiest thing to do when you don't know how the numeric data is stored in a character variable is:

Num_var = INPUT (Char_var, best32.);

This will output the character values as whole number.

Extracting Part of the String:

SUBSTR Function

We use SUBSTR function (Commonly pronounced "Sub-String"), to work with a specific position or positions of character within a defined character variable.

Syntax of Substr function: New_Var=Substr (Source, Position, N);

- Source -The first argument to this function is the input String.
- Position - The second argument is the starting position of where you want to extract your Sub-String
- N - The third, optional argument is the length of the Sub-String. If you omit the third argument, the function extracts a Sub-String from the input String up to the last non-blank character.

```
Data Sample;
Input String $ 1-15;
Site = Substr (String, 5, 4);
Patid = Substr (String, 10);
Datalines;
CTD-S101-P103
CTD-S102-P205
;
Run;
```

```
DATA Test;
String= 'SAS Clinical Programmer';
First=Substr (String, 1, 3);
Run;
```

> ***Written Test Question:*** What is the Length of the variable First in Test dataset?
>
> a) 8 b) 3 c) 200 d) 23

- If you did not include a LENGTH statement, SAS would still need to assign a length to the new variable. For this function, the default length is equal to the length of the first argument (Original String) to the function. (The work around for this issue is adding Length statement).

Using the SUBSTR Function on the Left-Hand Side of the Equal Sign:

- You can use this function to place characters in specific locations within a String by placing the SUBSTR function on the left hand side of the equal sign
- Suppose you have some systolic blood pressures (SBP) and diastolic blood pressures (DBP) in a SAS DATA set. You want to print out these values and star high values with an asterisk.

Here is a program that uses the SUBSTR function on the left of the equals sign to do that

```
Data pressure;
Input SBP DBP @@;
Datalines;
120 80 180 92 200 110
;
Run;

Data Pressure_Mod;
Set Pressure;
Length SBP_chk DBP_chk $ 6;
SBP_chk = PUT (SBP,3.);
DBP_chk = PUT (DBP,3.);
If SBP GT 160 then Substr (SBP_chk, 4, 1) = '*';
If DBP GT 90 then Substr (DBP_chk,4,1) = '*';
Run;
```

We first need to set the lengths of SBP_CHK and DBP_CHK to 4 (three spaces for the value plus one for the possible asterisk). Next, we use a PUT function to perform a numeric to character conversion.

It “writes out” the value of the first argument, according to the FORMAT specified in the second argument. By “write out” we actually mean assign the value to the variable on the left of the equal sign. The SUBSTR function then places an asterisk in the fourth position when a value of SBP is greater than 160 or a value of DBP is greater than 90.

SCAN Function:

Extracts a specified word from a character expression, where word is defined as the characters separated by a set of specified delimiters. The length of the returned variable is 200, unless previously defined.

Syntax: SCAN (character-value, n-word <,'delimiter-list'>)

- Character-value is any SAS character expression.
- N - Word is the nth “word” in the String.
- If n is greater than the number of words, the SCAN function returns a value that contains no characters.

- If n is negative, the character value is scanned from right to left.
- A value of zero is invalid.

```
Data Test;
String= 'SAS Clinical Programmer';
First=Scan (String, 1, 2);
Run;
```

By executing the above step, we created a dataset named test with a variable first. The value of the variable is Clinical.

> ***Written Test Question:*** What is the Length of the variable First in Test dataset?
>
> a) 8 b) 3 c) 200 d) 23

Functions That Substitute Letters or Words in Strings:

TRANSLATE Function can substitute one character for another in a String.

TRANWRD is more flexible—it can substitute a word or several words for one or more words.

TRANSLATE Function: To exchange Character value for another.

For example, you might want to change values 1–5 to the values A–E.

Translate function takes three arguments: The variable name, the character (or characters) you want in the Character String, and the character (or characters) you have in the character String.

Syntax: TRANSLATE (character-value, to-1, from-1 <,... to-n, from-n>);

- Character-value is any SAS character expression.
- To-n is a single character or a list of character values.
- From-n is a single character or a list of characters.
- Each character listed in from-n is changed to the corresponding value in to-n. If a character value is not listed in from-n, it will be unaffected.

TRANWRD Function:

To substitute one or more words in String with replacement word, words. It works like the find and replace feature of most word processors.

Syntax: TRANWRD (character-value, from-String, to-String)

- Character-value is any SAS character expression.
- From-String is one or more characters that you want to replace with the character or characters in the to-String.
- To-String is one or more characters that replace the entire from String.

USING LAG AND DIF FUNCTIONS:

The Retain statement holds the value of a variable across DATA step iterations and the LAG function returns the value of the variable from the previous observation. When used together, they allow the values of the previous and current observations to be compared so as to indentify consecutive occurrences of an event or condition, e.g., identifying consecutive abnormal glucose or blood pressure measurements over a specified period, when we need to relate the value of a variable in the current observation to the value of the same or another variable in the previous observation. The LAG function is a very useful tool for this purpose.

```
DATA Test;
Input Patid Visit Value @@;
Datalines;
101 1 200 101 2 210 101 3 220 101 4 225 101 5 220
102 1 300 102 2 290 102 3 295 102 4 270 102 5 250
;
Run;
Data Test_Mod;
SET Test;
L_Val = LAG (Value);
Chg_Prv = Value - L_Val;
Per_Chg = (Chg_Prv / L_Val)*100;
RUN;
```

The above code first calculates the Glucose value of the previous visit (L_Val) and the value difference (Chg_Prv) from one visit to the next. Then the percent increase is calculated from these two values. As expected, the first observation has missing values for all calculated variables. Here you can also use the DIF function to calculate the value difference. DIF works in the same way as LAG, except that it returns the difference between the value of the current observation and its lag, i.e.

- ✦ DIF (Value) = Value – LAG (Value).
- ✦ Per_Chg = (DIF (Value) / LAG (Value))*100

```
Data Test_R;
SET Test;
BY Patid Visit;
LAG_VAL = LAG (Value);
DIF_VAL = DIF (Value);
If First. Patid Then DO;
LAG_VAL = . ;
DIF_VAL = . ;
END;
Per_Chg = (DIF_VAL/LAG_VAL)*100;
Run;
```

Truncation Functions

FLOOR Function:

The FLOOR function takes numeric argument and returns the largest integer that is less than or equal to the argument.

CEIL Function:

The CEIL function returns the smallest integer that is greater than or equal to the argument.

INT Function:

The INT function returns the integer portion of the argument (truncates the decimal portion).

```
Data _Null_;
Val=32.261;
Flr_Val = FLOOR (Val);
Cil_Val = CEIL (Val);
Int_Val = INT (Val);
Put Flr_Val = Cil_Val = Int_Val =;
Run;
```

ROUND Function:

We use Round function to obtain the nearest value for the given value, we use this function frequently while rounding the lab result values. Usually we round the lab values to eighth decimal place.

```
Data Test;
Lab_Val= 37.826727628;
Rnd_Val1 = ROUND (Lab_Val);
Rnd_Val2 = ROUND (Lab_Val, .1);
Rnd_Val3 = ROUND (Lab_Val, .00000001);
Run;
```

Sample Statistics Functions

SUM Function – Returns the sum of non missing values

```
Data _Null_;
Sum_Val = SUM(9,8,.,9);
Put Sum_Val =;
Run;
```

MEAN Function – Returns the average of list of non missing values. We use this function to calculate Average, if the same parameter is collected for several times in the same visit in vitals and lab Datasets.

```
Data _Null_;
Avg_hr_M = Mean (86, 88, 87,.);
Avg_hr_Z =Mean (86, 88, 87, 0);
Put Avg_hr_M= Avg_hr_Z=;
Run;
```

- ***N Function*** - Counts the Number of non missing values in a list of values.
- ***NMISS Function*** - Counts the Number of missing values in a list of values.

The functions NMISS and N allow you to determine the number of missing values and non missing values, respectively, in the argument list.

```
Data Test;
NM_Val = NMISS (1,0,.,2,5,.);
N_Val = N (1,0,.,2,5,.);
Run;
```

DATE/TIME Functions

Date/Time functions are a set of functions that return portions of date time, date, or time values or convert numeric values for month, day and year or hour, minute and seconds into SAS date or time values. These functions are especially useful for extracting the date and time from a date time value or converting separate month, day and year values into a SAS date value.

SAS date variables are numeric variables containing integer values. The range of usable values goes from -138,061(January 01, 1582) to 6,589,335 (December 31, 20000). SAS time variables are also numeric variables. SAS times are a count of the number of seconds since midnight,1960 Jan01.

Date Functions:

TODAY Function: produces the current date in the form of a SAS date value, which is the number of days since January 1, 1960.

DATE Function: Returns the current date as a SAS date value.

TODAY, DATE Functions requires no arguments.

```
Data _Null_;
Tod_Val = TODAY ();
Dt_Val = DATE ();
Put Tod_Val = Dt_Val =;
Format Tod_Val ddmmyy10.;
Run;
```

WEEKDAY Function: WEEKDAY Function is to extract the day of the week from a SAS date value.(1=Sunday, ---, 7= Saturday)

Data _Null_;

DOB= '17apr1987'd;

*Dob_wk = WEEKDAY (DOB); *1(Sunday)-7(Saturday);*

Put Dob_wk =;

Run;

Extracting DAY, MONTH, and YEAR parts from a SAS date value:

We use ***DAY, MONTH, and YEAR Functions*** to Extract DAY, MONTH, and YEAR parts from a SAS date value. These functions are straightforward. They take SAS Date as the single argument and return the Day of the month, the month and the year.

Data Test;

ICDT=19758;

Dt_pt= DAY (Icdt);

Mn_pt = MONTH (Icdt);

Yr_pt= YEAR (Icdt);

Run;

DATETIME function will give the number of seconds elapsed from 1960jan01midnight

The date and or time elements (or 'parts') of a SAS datetime variable can be extracted using the ***DATEPART and TIMEPART functions.*** Suppose lab sample was collected from a patient at 5:45 p.m. on August 11, 2013, and a datetime variable (called LBDTM) is present in the database with this information. This value is the number of seconds between January 1, 1960 and 5:45 p.m. on August 11, 2013.

If only the date of collection is desired, DATE = DATEPART (LBDTM); returns the SAS date. Similarly, the time of collection can be obtained by: TIME = TIMEPART (LBDTM);

```
Data _Null_;
Dtm_Val = DATETIME ();
Tm_pt = TIMEPART (Dtm_Val);
Dt_pt = DATEPART (Dtm_Val);
Format Dt_pt ddmmyy10.;
Format Tm_pt Time8.;
Put Dtm_Val =;
Run;

Data Demo;
Input Id Birthyr @@;
Datalines;
101 1960 102 1975 103 1967
;
Run;
```

In the above Dataset only birth year is collected from subjects. Now our task is to assign day, month to those patients, so that data completes (Imputation), for this we use ***MDY function***.

```
Data YLP.DMADS;
Set YLP. Demog;
Birthdt=MDY (07, 01, Birthyr); *HARDCODE;
Format Birthdt date9.;
Run;
```

In the above program we assigned values July as Month and 01 as Day (As per SAP), so that they differ from the values stored in Database, this is known as Hard Coding. In hard coding we are explicitly changing the values of the Data so these values differs from the Database values. So, hard coding should be avoided as much as possible.

After performing hard coding we need to mention that in a separate document, the values and the variables that have been hard coded, name of the investigator and a comment HARDCODE in Capital Letters.

DHMS Function:

DHMS function is to create a SAS datetime value from a SAS date value and a value for the hour, minute, second.

Syntax: DHMS (Date, Hour, Minute, Second);

```
Data _Null_;
Ae_tm=DHMS ('05feb14'd, 09, 15, 18);
Put Ae_tm=;
Run;
```

INTCK Function:

Returns the number of time intervals in a given time span. The FROM and TO values are adjusted to the start of the stated INTERVAL. This means that '22mar1999'D will be seen as '01mar1999'd if the interval is 'MONTH' and as '01Jan 1999'd if the interval is 'YEAR'.

INTCK is to determine the number of time periods which have been crossed between two SAS date, time or datetime variables.

Syntax: INTCK ('Interval', from, to);

SAS Software allow users to declare a particular date or time as a constant without having to know the number of days from January 1, 1960 and/or the number of seconds since midnight. A date or time constant is declared by enclosing a date or time in single quotes, followed by the letter D and/or T to signify either date or time or DT to signify a datetime variable.

For example: ICDT = '04JUL2013'D will set the new variable ICDT equal to the number of days between January 1, 1960.

```
Data Test;
Birthdt='23Mar1980'D;
Icdt='18Jul2011'D;
Ageindy = INTCK ('Day', Birthdt, Icdt);
Ageinyr = Ageindy / 365.25;
Age = INT (Ageinyr);
Run;
```

INTNX Function:

Increments a date, time, or datetime value by a given time interval, and returns a date, time, or datetime value, It returns the date after specified number of intervals have passed. It creates a SAS date, time or datetime value that is a given number of time intervals from a starting value.

Syntax: INTNX ('Interval', From, To)

Suppose site wanted to send a remainder to the patients 4 days after the patient visit, reminding them to schedule a follow-up visit.

Rem_dt = INTNX ('Day',Visit1, 4);

Where Visit1 is a date variable representing first visit, the INTNX function will return values of Rem_dt which are the SAS date values four days past the patient's First Visit.

```
Data _Null_;
Visit1='20Sep2013'D;
Rem_dt = INTNX ('Day',Visit1,4);
Put Rem_dt = / Rem_dt date9.;
Run;

Data YLP.Dmads;
Merge YLP. Dmads YLP. Consent;
By Patid;
Run;

Data Dmads (Drop=Age_dy);
Set Dmads;
Age_dy=Intck ('Day', Birthdt, Icdt);
Ageyr =Int (Age_dy /365.25);
Run;
```

A Person, who never made a mistake, never tried anything new.

--Albert Einstein

STEP 8

UNDERSTANDING DATA STEP PROCESS AND PDV

When a program is been submitted in the Editor window, SAS checks the syntax of a program and reads the SAS statements and data, translates the program statements into executable machine code or intermediate code and Creates data sets, calls SAS Procedures, as requested, prints error messages in the Log and ends the job.

While Processing the SAS code, SAS Supervisor knows: The forms and types of statements that can be present in a DATA step, types of statements and the options that can be present in a PROC step.

To Process a program, the SAS Supervisor scans all the SAS statements and breaks each statement into words. (Tokens, tokenization happen in word scanner), each word is processed separately, when all the words in a step are processed, the step is executed. If the SAS Supervisor detects an error, then it flags the error at its location and prints an explanation.

Flow of action in a datastep

The Data Step consists of a group of SAS statements that begin with a Data statement. When you submit a Data step for execution, the complete syntax that makes up the Data Step is compiled, and the syntax is checked by SAS. If there is an error in the syntax, Processing is stopped and an error is output in the SAS Log. If the syntax is correct, then the statements are executed. In its simplest form, the Data step is a loop with an automatic output and return action at the end of each cycle.

When the syntax review is complete and no errors are found, SAS creates an Input Buffer, a Program Data Vector, and Descriptor Information.

- ***Input buffer:*** is a logical area in memory into which SAS reads each record of raw data when SAS executes an INPUT statement. Note that this buffer is created only when the DATA step reads raw data. (When the DATA step reads a SAS data set, SAS reads the data directly into the program data vector.)
- ***Program Data Vector (PDV):*** is a logical area in memory where SAS builds a data set, one observation at a time.
- ***Descriptor Information:*** is information that SAS creates and maintains about each SAS data set, including data set attributes and variable attributes.

All executable statements in the Data Step are processed once for each observation. If the input file contains raw data, SAS reads a record into the Input Buffer. SAS then reads the values in the Input Buffer and assigns the values to the appropriate variables in the Program Data Vector. SAS also calculates values for variables created by program statements, and writes these values to the Program Data Vector. When the program reaches the end of the Data Step syntax for each observation, SAS loops back to the beginning of the Data Step for the next observation.

Along with data set variables and computed variables, the PDV contains two ***automatic variables***, ***_N_ and _ERROR_.*** The *_N_* variable counts the number of times the DATA step begins to iterate. The *_ERROR_* variable signals the occurrence of an error caused by the data during execution. The value of _ERROR_ is either 0 (indicating no errors exist), or 1 (indicating that one or more errors have occurred). SAS does not write these variables to the output data set.

The program data vector is a storage place in memory that contains all of the variables encountered by the data step. The order of the variables in the program data vector is determined by when they are encountered. These variables may have indicators flagging them to be Kept, Dropped or Renamed. When the program runs, the program data vector contains the observation currently being processed. At the end of the step, the data are output according to the Drop, Keep, or Rename instructions encountered in the program.

At compilation time SAS creates the program data vector. The program data vector contains all the variables in the input data set and the variables created in the DATA step statements. Automatic variables are created automatically by the DATA step. Automatic variables are:

- Retained from one iteration of the DATA step to the next
- Not written to the output data set
- Cannot be kept, dropped, or renamed

Processing a DATA Step, a Walkthrough

```
Data Test (Drop= Pulse_M Pulse_N Pulse_E);
Put _all_;
Input Patid Sex $1. Trt$ Pulse_M Pulse_N Pulse_E ;
Avg_Pulse= (Pulse_M + Pulse_N+ Pulse_E)/3;
Put _all_;
Datalines;
101 F Placebo 88 100 94
102 M Active 100 96 104
103 F Active 78 84 81
;
Run;
```

- The input buffer and LPDV are set up at compile time and variables are added to the LPDV according to the way the INPUT statement and assignment statements are written.
- The purpose of the PUT __ALL__ statements will become apparent at execution time, when they will dump the contents of the LPDV to the LOG before and after the user-written statements are executed.
- The resulting LPDV contains all the information necessary for the descriptor portion of the SAS data set, Notice also that the LPDV contains information about which variables are written to the SAS data set being created, according to the default activities of DATA step Processing. These can be overridden through the use of DROP and KEEP statements or data set options. The LPDV also tracks which variables are retained.
- Note that all variables in the LPDV are initialized to missing at the beginning of each execution, except __N__ which is automatically retained.

- Note also that the DATA step will attempt to execute a fourth time, hence the dump of the LPDV to the LOG for __N__=4. The step will fail when the INPUT statement attempts to execute a fourth time since there is no more input data.
- When we apply the execution loop to the Processing of SAS data, we can observe the differences. The LPDV will continue to be displayed in the LOG via the PUT __ALL__ statements. The DATA step is reading data set 'Test' created in the previous step.

```
DATA R_test;
Put _all_;
Set Test;
Tot_rec+1;
Put _all_;
Run;
```

At compile time, the SET statement reads the descriptor portion of the input SAS data set in order to start building the LPDV. It retrieves the variables and their attributes. Additional variables will be added to the LPDV as their creation is encountered in subsequent SAS statements, in this case, the SUM statement to calculate TOT_REC.

Note that all variables in the LPDV will be retained. Patid, Sex, and Trt will be retained by default because they are being read in with a SET statement. TOT_REC is retained because it is the accumulator variable in a SUM statement (one of the features of the SUM statement is an implied retain).

Types of Errors in SAS

Syntax Error: Compilation phase

- Misspelled keyword
- Omitted semicolon
- Statement is not valid or it is used out of proper order

Execution Time Errors: Execution Phase

- Illegal mathematical operations
- Observations out of order for BY-group Processing

- An incorrect reference in an INFILE statement (for example, misspelling or otherwise incorrectly stating the external file)

Data Errors: Execution Phase

- Data in wrong columns
- Invalid data

Semantic Errors: Execution Phase

- Specifying the wrong number of arguments for a function
- Using a libref that has not yet been assigned
- Using a numeric variable name where only character variables are valid.

Common Automatic Variables

_*N*_*:* The number of times the Data step has iterated

***ERROR******:*** Indicates if an error has occurred in the data step or not. The value will be 0 if no errors occurred. It will be 1 if one or more errors occurred.

First. BY Variable and ***Last. BY Variable:*** These temporary variables always appear in pairs, One pair for each BY-variable on a BY statement. They have the value of 1(True) or 0(False) if the condition is true or false respectively. Temporary variables are created through the use of certain SAS options and statements, and like automatic variable, are not written to the output data set.

IN= variable: IN= is a data set option that indicates whether a particular data set has contributed to the current observation. The user specifies a variable name with the option that will have the value of 1 if the data set contributed to the observation or 0 if it did not.

END= Variable: END= is an option to the SET statement that indicates the end of the input data has been reached. The user defines a variable name that will have the value of 1 if the end of the data has been reached, 0 if it has not.

Only one END= can be specified on the SET statement. If multiple data sets are given in the SET statement, the END= variable will be set to 1 only when the last observation of the last data set has been read.

User defined variables can be assigned the value of automatic and temporary variables if it is necessary to have their values in the output data set.

STEP 9

MODIFYING SAS DATASETS

SOP (Standard Operating Procedure) states that Temporary Datasets should be as concise as possible and should only contain the variables and observations necessary for the program to execute without error.

This can be achieved by using WHERE, KEEP and DROP statements when accessing datasets. Redundant variables and observations should be removed from datasets as early as possible. This will result in programs running faster and will make the datasets easier to view.

In general, it is far more efficient to use WHERE, KEEP and DROP statements when inputting a dataset rather than Outputting a dataset - this avoids unnecessary Processing of unwanted variables.

Conditional Processing

Quite often we need to Process DATA based on certain conditions, for this we use conditional Processing. Conditional Processing can be done by many ways:

- IF
- WHERE
- SELECT OTHERWISE

1. ***Subsetting IF statement:*** Continues processing only those observations that meet the condition of the specified expression.

Syntax of sub setting IF: IF Condition;

DATA Demog_f;

Set YLP.Demog;

IF Sex=1;

Run;

2. ***Conditional IF statement:*** The IF statement evaluates the logical expression and THEN conditionally executes the THEN statement. The sub statement that follows the THEN keyword is executed when the logical expression result is non missing and nonzero.

Syntax: IF logic-expression THEN statement;

```
DATA Demog_f;
Set YLP.Demog;
IF Sex=1 THEN OUTPUT;
Run;
```

3. ***Multiple conditional IF Statement:***

```
DATA Aemiss Aemild Aemod Aesev;
Set YLP.Events;
IF Aesev = 1 THEN Output Aemild;
IF Aesev=2 THEN Output Aemod;
IF Aesev=3 THEN Output Aesev;
IF Aesev=. THEN Output Aemiss;
Run;
```

In the above step we created four Datasets based on the four different conditions.

Creating a flag variable based on conditions:

```
Data YLP.Dmads;
Set YLP.Dmads;
If 0 <= AGEYR < 65 then AGEGRP = '< 65 years';
Else if AGEYR >= 65 then AGEGRP = '>= 65 years';
Run;
```

```
DATA Events;
Length Aesevlnm $10;
Set YLP.Events;
IF Aesev = 1 THEN Aesevlnm='Mild';
IF Aesev=2 THEN Aesevlnm='Moderate';
IF Aesev=3 THEN Aesevlnm='Severe';
IF Aesev=. THEN Aesevlnm= 'Miss';
Run;
```

4. Mutually exclusive conditional IF Statement:

```
DATA Ae_Mild Ae_Mod Ae_Sev Miss;
Set YLP.Events;
Put _All_;
IF Aesev = 1 THEN Output Ae_Mild;
ELSE IF Aesev=2 THEN Output Ae_Mod;
ELSE IF Aesev=3 THEN Output Ae_Sev;
ELSE Output Miss;
Run;
```

- SAS evaluates the expression in an IF-THEN statement to produce a result that is non-zero, zero, or missing. A non-zero and non missing result causes the expression to be true. A result of zero or missing causes the expression to be false.
- IF the conditions that are specified in the IF clause are met, the IF-THEN statement executes a SAS statement for observations that are read from a SAS Data set, for records in an external file, or for computed values.
- An optional ELSE statement gives an alternative action IF the THEN clause is not executed. The ELSE statement, IF used, must immediately follow the IF-THEN statement
- Using IF-THEN statements without the ELSE statement causes SAS to evaluate all IF-THEN statements. Using IF-THEN statements with the ELSE statement causes SAS to execute IF-THEN statements until it encounters the first true statement.

5. IF Statement with DO loop

IF condition THEN

DO;

Action1;

Action2;

-----;

END;

6. Select Statement: (Select - Otherwise):

It executes one of several statements or groups of statements. The SELECT statement begins a SELECT group. SELECT groups contain WHEN statements that identify SAS statements that are executed when a particular condition is true. Use at least one WHEN statement in a SELECT group. An optional OTHERWISE statement specifies a statement to be executed IF no WHEN condition is met. An END statement ends a SELECT group. Null statement that are used in WHEN statements cause SAS to recognize a condition as true without taking further action. Null statements that are used in OTHERWISE statements prevent SAS from issuing an error message when all WHEN conditions are false.

7. Where statement:

Understanding the WHERE Statement:

- ✦ The WHERE statement is the simplest way to subset DATA.
- ✦ This statement specifies the observations to include in the analysis.
- ✦ SAS excludes observations that do not meet the criteria in the WHERE statement.
- ✦ The WHERE statement can help your programs Run faster because SAS uses only the observations that meet the criteria in the WHERE statement. This advantage can be very helpful with large DATA sets.
- ✦ The WHERE statement uses unformatted values of variables, so you need to specify unformatted values in the statement.
- ✦ You can use the WHERE statement with any SAS Procedure.
- ✦ The WHERE statement allows all of the usual arithmetic and comparison operators. For example, you can add, subtract,

multiply, and divide in the statement. You can specify comparison operators like equal to, not equal to, greater than, and so on.

- The WHERE statement has special operators that are available only in the statement. Three operators that are especially useful are IS MISSING, BETWEEN-AND, and CONTAINS.

The general form of the statement to specify DATA to include in a Procedure is shown below:

Syntax: WHERE expression;

Expression is a 1) Combination of variables, 2) Comparison operators, 3) Values that specify the observations to include in the Procedure.

BY-Group Processing

- By group Processing is a method of processing observations from one or more SAS DATA sets that are grouped or ordered by values of one or more common variables.
- The most common use of BY-group Processing in the DATA step is to combine two or more SAS DATA sets by using the BY statement with a SET, MERGE .
- BY variable: a variable or variables by which the DATA set is sorted.

SAS identifies the beginning and end of a BY group by creating two temporary variables for each BY variable:

- FIRST. Variable
- LAST. Variable

The value of these variables is either 0 or 1. SAS sets the value of First. Variable to 1 when it reads the first observation in a BY group, and sets the value of LAST.Variable to 1 when it reads the last observation in a BY group.

The FIRST. Variable and LAST. Variable values indicate whether an observation is:

- The first in a BY group
- The last in a BY group
- Neither the first nor the last in a BY group
- Both first and last, as is the case when there is only one observation in a BY group.

These temporary variables are available for DATA step programming but are not added to the Output DATA set. Use these temporary variables to conditionally Process sorted, grouped DATA.

There is a three-step Process for accumulating totals:

- Set the accumulating variable to 0 at the start of each BY group.
- Increment the accumulating variable with a sum statement (automatically retains).
- Output only the last observation of each BY group.

```
Data Demog;
Input Id Gender$ Race @@;
Datalines;
101 m 1 102 f 2 103 m 3 104 m 2 105 f 1
106 f 2 107 m 1 108 m 1 109 f 1 110 f 3
;
Run;

Proc Sort Data=Demog out=Demsrt;
By gender;
Run;
```

Counting subjects by gender

```
Data Gen_cnt;
Set Demsrt;
By Gender;
IF First. Gender THEN Count=0;
Count+1;
IF Last. Gender;
Run;

Data Demog;
Input id Trt $ Gender$ Race @@;
```

Datalines;

101 active m 1 102 placebo f 2 103 active m 1 104 active m 2 105 active f 1

106 placebo f 2 107 active m 1 108 placebo f 3 109 placebo m 2 110 active f 1

;

Run;

Tasks:

TASK: Write a program to create the following Information: ✦ To count number of subjects assigned to specific treatment. ✦ To count number of subject assigned to specific treatment gender wise. ✦ Count the number of subjects as per trt and race

Data Test;

Input Patid Trt Ae $ @@;

Datalines;

101 1 YES 102 2 NO 103 1 NO 104 1 YES 105 2 YES

106 2 YES 107 2 NO 108 2 YES 109 1 NO 110 2 YES

;

Run;

Task: Count the number of subjects assigned to Trt 1 and got Adverse Events

Differences between IF and WHERE:

WHERE conditions are applied before the DATA enters the input buffer while IF conditions are applied after the DATA enters the program DATA vector.

This is the reason why the WHERE condition is faster because not all observations have to be read and because it can only be applied on variables that exist in the input DATA set.

Summary of Key Differences between WHERE and IF Conditions:

1. Either WHERE or IF Conditions can be used

- ✦ Using on variables in DATA set
- ✦ Using Set, Merge statement IF within the DATA step

2. Must use IF Condition

- ✦ Accessing raw DATA file using Input statement
- ✦ Using automatic variables such as _N_, First. By, Last. By
- ✦ Using newly created variables in DATA set
- ✦ In combination with DATA set options such as OBS =,FIRSTOBS =

3. Must use WHERE Condition

- ✦ Using special operators such as ‘Like’ or ‘Contains’
- ✦ Directly using any SAS Procedure
- ✦ When Subsetting as a DATA set option
- ✦ When Subsetting using Proc SQL

Points to remember:

- ✦ Accessing raw DATA file using INPUT statement – Use IF statement
- ✦ Using automatic variables such as _N_, FIRST.BY, LAST.BY – Use IF statement
- ✦ Using newly created variables in DATA set – Use IF statement
- ✦ Using special operators such as LIKE or CONTAINS – Use WHERE statement
- ✦ Directly using any SAS Procedures – Use WHERE statement

```
DATA Demog;
Input Id Gender$ Race @@;
Datalines;
101 m 1 102 f 2 103 m 3 104 m 2 105 f 1
106 f 2 107 m 1 108 m 1 109 f 1 110 f 3
;
Run;
```

Using variables in dataset, using SET, MERGE statement IF within the DATA step –

Although WHERE or IF statement can be used, for better performance, use the WHERE statement.

In this example, the DATA step contains a WHERE statement based on a variable in the demog Data set. The SET statement is used to access the DEMOG Data set. The records in the new Data set, PAT_F, will contain only those records that meet the WHERE condition.

```
Data Pat_F;
Set Demog;
Where Gender = 'f';
Run;
```

We Can use WHERE condition because GENDER variable is a DATA set variable, WHERE condition requires all DATA set variables.

In this case, you can apply the IF statement instead of the WHERE statement to get the same results. Note that in the basic form, the syntax of WHERE and IF statements are the same except for the keyword.

```
Data Pat_M;
Set Demog;
IF Gender = 'm';
Run;
```

What would happen IF you incorrectly specified the IF statement by mixing a numeric variable in a character expression as shown below:

```
Data test;
Set demog;
IF RACE = '2';
Run;
```

- With IF conditions, SAS will automatically converts variable types.
- With WHERE conditions, however, SAS does not automatically convert variable types. It generates an ERROR message because operator requires compatible variables.

```
Data Test1;
Set DEMOG;
Where race = '2';
Run;
```

ERROR: Where clause operator requires compatible variables.

Using automatic variables such as _N_, FIRST.BY, LAST.BY – Must use IF statement

When specifying a condition based on automatic or temporary variables within a DATA step, you must use the IF statement. In this example, the DEMOG DATA set is sorted by the GENDER variable. The DATA step uses the IF statement to keep the FIRST.GENDER record, because these temporary variables exist only in the program DATA vector. Variables in the WHERE statement must exist in the DATA set. Note that IF the dot is missing between the FIRST and NAME, THEN SAS creates the FIRST variable as a numeric variable, converts the NAME variable from a character to a numeric variable and THEN expects an operator between FIRST and NAME.

```
Proc Sort Data = Demog Out=Demsrt;
By Gender;
Run;
```

Use IF condition because Gender is the BY variable

Data DEMSRT2;

Set DEMSRT;

By Gender;

IF First. Gender;

Run;

As you can see below, there is only one record for each GENDER. This meets the subset condition to keep only the first record for each unique value of the SUBJECT GENDER.

Using newly created variables in DATA set – Must use IF statement

When specifying conditions based on variables created within the same Data step, you must use the IF statement because that variable exists only in the program Data vector. In this example, the GENNUM variable is created from the GENDER variable. The records in the new Dataset, TEST3, will contain only those records that meet the IF condition.

Data Test3;

Set Demog;

IF Gender = 'f' THEN Gen_num = 1;

ELSE IF gender = 'm' THEN Gen_num = 2;

IF Gen_num = 2;

Run;

All records meet the condition which requires the Gen_num variable to equal 2 will be created in the data set. IF you replace the IF statement with a WHERE statement, Then you will get the following error message. This is because the WHERE statement requires variables to exist in the demog Data set.

Data test3;

Set Demog;

IF GENDER = 'f' THEN Gen_num = 1;

ELSE IF gender = 'm' THEN Gen_num = 2;

Where Gen_num = 2;

Run;

ERROR: Variable Gen_num is not on file WORK.Demog.

Using special operators such as LIKE or CONTAINS – Must use WHERE statement

IF you could not remember the exact spelling of Event's name, then you can take advantage of special operators such as LIKE or CONTAINS in the WHERE condition. Notice that this syntax is unique to the WHERE statement. In addition, when working with character variables consider case sensitivity by using the UPCASE function and are aware of embedded blanks.

DATA test4;

Set YLP.Events;

Where Socterm contains 'gast';

Run;

Directly using any SAS Procedure or as a DATA set option – Must use WHERE condition

A big advantage of using the WHERE condition is the ability to apply the subset condition directly in SAS Procedures. This approach not only avoids a DATA step to first subset the Data set, but also prevents the need to create a separate Data set.

Proc Print DATA = Demog;

Where Gender = 'f' or Race= 1;

Run;

If you replace the WHERE statement with an IF statement, THEN you will get the following error message. IF statement is not valid outside the DATA step. When possible, specify WHERE statements in SAS Procedures to avoid unnecessary Data step Processing.

Proc Print Data = DEMOG;

IF GENDER = 'f' or RACE= 1;

Run;

ERROR: Statement is not valid or it is used out of proper order.

Note that multiple WHERE conditions are not cumulative unless the '***ALSO***' keyword is used. By default, the most recent WHERE condition replaces the previous WHERE condition.

```
Proc Print Data = Demog;
Where Gender = 'f';
Where also Race= 1;
Run;
```

WHERE dataset Option and condition may be applied for cumulative effect.

```
Proc Print Data = Demog (Where= (GENDER = 'f'));
Where Race= 1;
Run;
```

When applying multiple IF conditions within a DATA step, however, the conditions become cumulative.

```
DATA Test5;
Set Demog;
IF gender = 'f';
IF race = 2;
Run;
```

In addition, mixing IF and WHERE conditions within a DATA step also become cumulative.

```
DATA Test6;
Set Demog;
IF gender = 'f';
Where race = 2;
Run;
```

Understanding Do - Loops

The term 'loop' describes any control structure that causes a set of programming logic to be executed iteratively

Every DO–loop consists of three parts: beginning, middle, and end.

Syntax of Do - Loop

```
DO Index = start <TO stop> <BY increment> <WHILE (expression)
| UNTIL (expression)> ;
<SAS Code>
End;
```

Start is the top of the loop; it is here that an index variable will be specified and the exit conditions of the loop will be established.

Increment is the code that the loop will iterate over; this code can be static or modified in part by the iterations of the loop.

Expression is the "end" of the loop; however, many people like to refer to this as the bottom rather than the end because the test to exit can be anywhere within the DO-loop.

DO Statement:

The DO statement designates a group of statements that are to be executed as a unit.

The simplest form of the DO loop is:

```
DO;
Statement1;
Statement2;
    . . .
END;
```

We have two basic types of DO-loops, ***1) Implicit and 2) Explicit***

Within these two main types, there are two subtypes, ***1) Iterative and 2) Infinite***

The only implicit DO-loop in SAS that can be controlled to some extent is the DATA step internal loop, which is infinite. Explicit DO-loops can be iterative or infinite.

Implicit Loops:

An implicit loop is nothing more than a loop performed by the language without the programmer specifically writing it in the code.

The need for the DATA step to read each observation, whether that observation comes from an external file or SAS DATA set, is implied by the fact that a DATA step is being used by the programmer. Since the DATA step either cannot determine the number of loops to perform or cannot do so efficiently, the implied DO-loop is an infinite one, with orders to exit the looping action when there is no more DATA to be read.

Iterative DO Loops:

The iterative DO loop executes the statements between DO and END repetitively based on the value of an index variable

Syntax of Iterative do-loop: DO index-variable = start TO stop;

IF all this sounds confusing that is because DO iterative is also the most flexible of the DO-loops with a great many possible applications.

```
DATA One;
      Do I = 1 To 10;
            Output;
      End;
Run;
DATA Two;
Put 'Before:' _All_ ;
Set One;
Put 'After:' _All_;
Run ;
```

DO Iterative:

The DO Iterative is the most basic type of DO-loop in SAS. It iterates over the values given in its index variable. This can take many forms:

- ✦ List of numeric or character values separated by comma;
- ✦ A range given by a start value, an ending value and a by value;
- ✦ Some combination of the previously stated and a WHILE or UNTIL condition.

To clarify let's look at some examples.

DO Iterative Example1

```
DATA Test1;
    Do I = 1, 2, 3;
      Put I=;
    End;
Run;
```

DO Iterative Example2:

```
DATA Test2;
      Do I = 'A', 'B', 'C';
         Put I=;
      End;
Run;
```

- In the above two examples we see that the DO Iterative will loop for every value in a list that is given to the index variable. It does not matter whether that list is numeric or character. What do matter is that all the values in that list are of the same type. This is due to the fact that the index variable becomes an actual variable in the DATA set, thus it must follow the rules of SAS variables in that it cannot be both a numeric and character at the same time.
- When working with a character list, be sure all values are of the same length; you can ensure this by making sure you have the same number of spaces between parentheses or by using a LENGTH statement to set the value of the index variable to the length of the longest value in your list.

Syntax of Iterative do-loop:

DO Index-variable = Start TO Stop;

```
DATA _Null_;
        Do I = 1 To 10 By 2;
           Put I=;
        End;
Put I=;
Run;
```

- From the log we see that a value of 11 after the loop is finished. After the loop where the value of I is 9, control passes back to the top of the loop, I is incremented by two to reach 11. That is tested and found to be greater than the stop value of 10 so the loop stops. However, the value of I is now 11 and not 9, the last value before it would be greater than 10 or equal to 10 as the stop value. This underscores the importance of knowing specifically what is happening before using the index variables later in code.

Try the following codes and check the datasets for your clarity:

DATA Do_Lp1; *DO Id=1 to 10;* *END;* *Run;*	*DATA Do_Lp2;* *DO Id=1 to 10;* *Output;* *END;* *Run;*
DATA Do_Lp3; *DO Id=1 to 10 by 4;* *Output;* *END;* *Run;*	*DATA Do_Lpx;* *DO Id=1 to 10 by 4;* *END;* *Output;* *Run;*
DATA Do_Lpy; *DO Id=1 to 16 by 5;* *Output;* *END;* *Output;* *Run;*	*DATA Do_Lpz;* *DO Id=1 to 20 by 10;* *Output;* *END;* *Run;*

Using UNTIL and WHILE Clauses

You can add either an UNTIL clause or a WHILE clause to your DO statements.

DO Index-variable = start TO stop |;

- The UNTIL expression is evaluated after the statements in the DO loop have executed, and the WHILE expression is evaluated before the statements in the DO loop have executed.
- The statements in a DO UNTIL loop are always executed at least once, but the statements in a DO WHILE loop will not execute even once IF DO WHILE expression is false.

DO WHILE Clause

- The DO While, unlike the basic DO Iterative, is an infinite loop with an exit condition. Thus IF the exit criteria is never met the loop will continue until stopped by something outside the looping code. The exit criteria of a DO While loop assumes a true condition and looks for when that true condition becomes false in order to stop the looping Process.

- The DO WHILE loop tests for this exit criteria at the top of the loop. Thus, IF the criteria are false the first time it is tested THEN the loop will not iterate at all.

DO While Example #1

```
DATA _Null_;
I = 0;
        Do While (I < 10);
            Put I=;
        I + 1;
        End;
Run;
```

- Here our exit criteria states when the value of I is equal to the value of 10 the loop stops.
- We set the index variable's initial value to 0, (this is called priming the loop), the exit criteria test is done and found to be true so the loop iterates.
- The value of I is written to the log and THEN its value is incremented by 1.
- Control passes to the top of the Loop; the test is performed and again found to be true.
- The steps are repeated until the value of I is equal to the stop criteria thresh hold of 10.

DO While Example #2

```
DATA _Null_;
I = 11;
        Do While (I<10);
        Put I=;
        I + 1;
        End;
Run;
```

- Here we primed the loop's initial value to 11 and one can see from the log that no values were written out.

- The initial test was made and the exit criteria expression was resolved to false.
- Thus the DO while loop did not execute.

DO While Example #3

We saw in the first example that the loop apparently iterated 10 times; however what exactly is the end value of index variable I in that example?

```
DATA _Null_;
I = 0;
        Do While (I<10);
        Put 'Inside Loop:' I=;
        I + 1;
        End;
Put 'Outside Loop:' I=;
Run;
```

- We see from the log that the ending value of I is 10.
- The loop initially iterated as expected, the last value from inside the loop printed to the log is 9 which is less than the value of 10 as set in our loop's exit criteria.
- However, after the loop where I with value of 9 is printed to the log, the value of I gets incremented one more time to 10.
- Control is passed to the top of the loop, the value is checked one last time and the exit criterion is shown to be false.

DO UNTIL Clause

The DO Until loop, like the DO While, is an infinite loop with set exiting criteria.

Unlike the DO While, the DO UNTIL exit condition is assumed false and the loop stops only when the criteria becomes true.

Yet another difference is that it tests for this exit condition at the bottom of the loop.

Thus, it will always iterate at least once.

DO Until Example #1

```
DATA _Null_;
I =0;
        Do Until (I >10);
        Put I=;
        I + 1;
        End;
Run;
```

- We see from the above example that the loop starts with a value of 0 on its first iteration and continues until the value of I is 10. The value of I for the first iteration of the loop is printed out to the log, THEN incremented by 1, THEN the test for the exit condition is performed and finally control is passed to the top of the loop.
- Once the value of I is incremented to a value of 11, when the condition is tested and found to be true, the loop stops iterating.

DO Until Example #2

```
DATA _Null_ ;
I = 11;
Do Until (I>10);
Put I=;
I + 1;
End;
Run;
```

- In this example we see that though we set the initial value of I to 11 the DO Until loop does still execute one time.
- Remember that because this type of loop tests at the bottom, it will iterate one time regardless of whether the exit condition is true or not so we see the initial value of I written to the log.

```
DATA _Null_ ;
I = 0;
Do Until (I >10);
Put 'Inside Loop: ' I=;
I + 1;
End;
Put 'After Loop: ' I=;
Run;
```

- Just like in the DO While loop we see that the last value of I is indeed 11. This makes intuitive sense given that our stated exit condition was to stop loop when I became greater than 10.

Written Test Questions:

Question 1: *DATA Test1;* *x=6;* *Do while (x le 6);* *x+1;* *End;* *Run;*	***Question 2:*** *DATA Test2;* *Do while (n lt 6);* *n+1;* *End;* *Run;*
Question 3: *DATA Test3;* *Do until (x gt 6);* *x+1;* *End;* *Run;*	***Question4:*** *DATA Test7;* *I =0;* *Do While (I <= 10);* *I + 1;* *End;* *Run;*
Question5: *DATA Test5;* *n=3;* *Do while (n<5);* *Put n=;* *n+1; Output;* *End; Output;* *Run;*	***Question6:*** *DATA Test6;* *I = 0;* *Do While (I<10);* *Output;* *I + 1;* *End;* *Run;*

Question 7: *DATA Test4;* *n=3;* *Do while (n<5);* *Put n=;* *n+1; Output;* *End;* *Run;*	***Question8:*** *DATA Test8;* *I = 5;* *Do Until (I =>10);* *Put I=;* *I + 1;* *Output;* *End;* *Run;*

Debugging

Debugging is a Process of finding out the program logic and the number of iterations getting executed in a data step. While using debug option SAS opens two windows:

- Debugger Log
- Debugger source, which will help us to understand the back end Process of iterations

```
Data Test / DEBUG;
        DO I= 1 to 20 by 7;
        Output;
        END;
Run;
```

Creating User Generated Log Messages

When we are checking for the completeness and validity of the data we can create user generated log messages, while creating user generated log messages we split the word into two parts so that they would not appear in Red, Green, Blue colors in the log window.

```
DATA _Null_;
Set YLP.Demog;
        If Sex = . Then
Put "Err" "or: Missing Gender Info:" Patid= Sex=;
Run;
```

RETAIN Statement

- Causes a variable that is created by an INPUT or assignment statement to retain its value from iteration of the DATA step to the next.
- This is in contrast to the default DATA step behavior, which is, Without a RETAIN statement, SAS automatically sets variables that are assigned values by an INPUT or assignment statement to missing before iteration of the DATA step.
- A starting value is assigned to the retained variable.
- The variables being retained are not initialized with missing values at the top of the cycle, but retain their previous value.
- The RETAIN statement specifies variables whose values are not set to missing at the beginning of each iteration of the DATA step, causing SAS to hold the value from one iteration of the DATA step to the next.
- Only variables not in the input DATA sets can be retained.
- IF we can create a variable to retain a patient's baseline weight on every record, we can calculate the change from baseline, by subtracting baseline weight from current weight at any visit for which weight was measured.
- Another use of RETAIN might involve retaining the most recent visit's weight, so we can use this value in the case that weight was not measured for a particular visit.

Syntax for the RETAIN statement:

RETAIN Variable_name <Initial Value>;

- RETAIN Y 0; -- Assigns the variable Yan initial value of 0.
- RETAIN Y . ; -- Assigns the variable Y an initial value of . (missing), Y will be written to DATA set.
- RETAIN Y; -- Also Assigns the variable Y an initial value of . (missing), Y will not be written to DATA set unless an initial value is assigned elsewhere.

This example illustrates a number of different scenarios.

```
DATA one;
a = 1; b = 1; c=5;Output;
a = 1; b = .; c=5;Output;
a = 1; b = .; c=5;Output;
Run;

DATA two;
d = 0; e = 0; Output;
d = 1; e = 0; Output;
d = 2; e = 0; Output;
Run;

DATA Three;
Set One Two;
Retain a 5 b;
IF _n_ = 1 THEN f = 0;
a + 1;
b = b + 1;
e + 1;
f = f + 1;
g + 1;
Run;
```

Variable A – input from DATA set ONE, variable is retained (explicitly and implicitly), value is calculated. The RETAIN, both explicit and implicit have no obvious effect on the first three observations because the value comes from the input DATA set.

When the second input DATA set is encountered, the value is set to missing and the effects of the RETAIN become evident. At observation 4, the value is set to missing due to its non-existence in the second input DATA set, the sum statement calculates the value on observation 4: missing (input value) + 1 = 1 and a new value is Output.

Variable B – input from DATA set ONE; variable is retained; value is calculated. Though the variable is explicitly retained, the value is not retained from the first observation because the variable comes from one or more of the input DATA sets.

Variable C – input from DATA set ONE. At observation 4 the variable is reset to missing when the second input DATA set is encountered.

Variable D – input from DATA set TWO. The variable exists in the first three Output observations, though it has a missing value. The variable values are introduced to the program DATA vector starting at observation 4.

Variable E – input from DATA set TWO; implicitly retained by the sum statement; value is calculated. The sum statement calculates the value on observation 1: missing (input value) + 1 = 1. At the second observation the value is incremented by one, and again in the third observation. At observation 4, the value is set to 0 by the second input DATA set. The value is THEN incremented and Output. At observation 5 the value is again set to 0 by the second input DATA set, incremented, and Output.

Variable F – value is initialized when _N_ is 1; value is calculated. The variable is not on an input DATA set, and it is not retained, therefore, at observation 2, it is reset to missing. The statement used to increment the variable F is not a sum statement, therefore, when the value is reset to missing at observation 2, the result of the addition is missing.

Variable G – value is calculated; implicitly retained by the sum statement. The value is not reset to missing at observation 4 because the value is retained and is not on an input DATA set.

Summary of some of the rules of Retain Statement:

- Retaining a variable of an input dataset has no effect. Their values will be set by the input dataset.
- At the start of iteration of the DATA step, non-retained variables created in a DATA step are set to missing.
- Variables created with a sum statement are automatically retained.
- IF a variable name is specified in the RETAIN statement with no initial value and receives no value from Processing, the variable is not written to the Dataset, and a note stating that the variable is uninitialized is written to the SAS log.

Using Retain statement in Calculating Change from Baseline Value:

```
Data Vital;
Set YLP.Vitals;
Where Vstest in ('sys', 'dia', 'hrt');
Run;

Proc sort data=Vital Out=Vitalsrt;
By Patid Vstest visid;
Run;

Data YLP. CFB (Keep=Patid Vstest Baseline Change Pct_chg );
Set Vitalsrt;
By Patid Vstest visid;
**** CARRY FORWARD BASELINE RESULTS.;
Retain Baseline;
If First. Vstest then Baseline = .;
If Visid = 3 then Baseline = Vsrn;
else if Visid > 3 then
        Do;
            Change = Vsrn - Baseline;
            Pct_Chg = ((Vsrn - Baseline) /Baseline )*100;
        End;
If Last. Vstest ;
Run;
```

Array

SAS Clinical programmers use arrays to simplify their code, which results in programs that are frequently more efficient and less error-prone. When we want to Process multiple variables, want take multiple actions on multiple variables, more statements are required. As a result, the Process becomes more tedious and error prone. Arrays can be used to perform this Process with far fewer statements.

A SAS array is a convenient way of temporarily identifying a group of variables for Processing within a data step. Once the array has been defined the programmer is now able to perform the same tasks for a series of related variables, the array elements.

It makes sense to use arrays when there are repetitive values that are related and the programmer needs to iterate though most of them. The combination of arrays and do loops in the data step lend incredible power to programming. The most important aspect of arrays is that they will allow you to save time and typing by avoiding repetitious data step coding. Repetitious code occurs when you find yourself coding the same line over and over again with the only change being the variable name. You achieve code simplicity by grouping the variables into an array and performing array Processing.

Array Processing involves:

- Grouping variables into arrays.
- Performing an action, and then repeating the action.
- Selecting the current variable to be acted upon.

Array Processing is enhanced by using a DO loop. The DO loop is used to tell the SAS system to perform the same action several times.

To use arrays in SAS code, first make sure that you understand the basic syntax of the SAS ARRAY statement.

Syntax of array:

Array Array-name {n} <$> <length> array-elements < (initial-values)>;

Where

- Array-name – Any valid SAS name
- n – Number of elements within the array
- $ - Indicates the elements within the array are character type variables
- Length – A common length for the array elements
- Elements – List of SAS variables to be part of the array
- Initial values – Provides the initial values for each of the array elements.

Variables that are associated with an array have certain characteristics:

- All variables that are associated with an array must be of the same type, either character or numeric. As a result, arrays are typically referred to as either character arrays or numeric arrays.
- Variables that are associated with an array do not have to be already existing variables. If they do not exist within a program data vector (PDV) when the ARRAY statement is compiled, SAS creates them for you.
- Variables that are not previously defined as character variables will default to numeric variables unless they are defined as character variables within the ARRAY statement. To define character variables within the ARRAY statement, place a dollar sign ($) after the brackets and before any of the variables.

Arrays are of Two Types: 1. Static Array 2. Dynamic Array

```
Data Chol;
Input Visit Ldl Idl Hdl;
Datalines;
1 45 63 .
2 . 75 150
3 62 . 98
4 . . 67
;
Run;
```

1. Static Array: Fixed Size, Simplest Type of Array

```
Data Sta_Ary;
Set Chol;
Array _Ch {3} LDL IDL HDL;
Do I= 1 to 3;
If _Ch{I}=. Then _Ch{I}= 0;
End;
Run;
```

2. Dynamic Array:

- No Fixed Size,
- Grow or shrink with different data automatically
- * is used to represent the array size
- The function DIM (array name) returns the number of elements in that array

```
Data Dyn_Ary (drop=I);
Set Chol;
Array Ch[*] _All_;
Do I= 1 to dim (Ch);
If Ch{I}=. then Ch{I}=0;
End;
Run;
```

Differences between static and Dynamic Array:

- We did not mention the No. of array elements (*)
- We do not know the number of variables to Process (_All_)
- We specified DIM (Array Name) instead of Number of Iterations (upper Limit)

Applications of arrays in SAS Clinical Programming

- LOCF (Last Observation Carry Forward)
- Visit sequence (count consecutive days)
- To search a specified value
- Convert missing values to zero

Replacing missing values with certain other values for multiple variables;

```
Data Chol;
Input Visit Ldl Idl Hdl;
Datalines;
1 45 63 .
2 . 75 150
3 62 . 98
4 . . 67
;
Run;

Data Chol_Mod (Drop=I);
Set Chol;
Array _Ch{3} Ldl Idl Hdl;
DO I = 1 to 3;
If _Ch{i}=. Then _ch{i}=999;
END;
Run;

DATA Dyn_Ary;
Length A B C D E $ 1;
Input A B C D E X Y;
Datalines;
M f P p D 1 2
m f m F M 3 4
;
Run;
```

If we want to Process only the character variables, since we do not know the number of variables we use DIM function. DIM function: Returns the number of elements in an array.

```
DATA Ary_UP;
SET  Dyn_Ary;
ARRAY _Cha [*] _CHARACTER_;
DO I = 1 TO DIM(_Cha);
_Cha [I] = UPCASE(_Cha[I]);
END;
Drop I;
Run;
```

Believe you can, you're half way there.

--Theodore Roosevelt

STEP 10

STATISTICAL CONCEPTS

Biostatistics: It is the science which deals with development and application of the most appropriate methods for the:

- Collection of data.
- Presentation of the collected data.
- Analysis and interpretation of the results.
- Making decisions on the basis of such analysis

Biostatistics—the theory and techniques for collecting, describing, analyzing, and interpreting health data, When the data analyzed are derived from the biological science and medicine.

Statistics is the studies of how to collect, organize, analyze, and interpret numerical information from data.

Statistics is the art/science of summarizing data, Clinical investigations usually involve collecting a lot of data. But, at the end of your trial, what we really want is a "punch-line"

- Did the new treatment work?
- Are the two groups being compared the same or different?
- Is the new method more precise than the old method?

Common statistical terms

Population: A population is a universe of entities to be characterized, but is too vast to study in its entirety.

Example:

- Patients with mild-to-moderate hypertension
- Obese teenagers
- Adult, insulin-dependent, diabetic patients.

Sample: A sample is a group of units selected from a larger group (the population). By studying the sample it is hoped to draw valid conclusions about the larger group.

Parameter: is a summary measure that describes a characteristic of the population.

Statistics: is a summary measure computed from a sample to describe a characteristic of the population.

Data: the facts and figures to be –Collected, Summarized, Analyzed, Interpreted.

- The raw material of Statistics is data.
- We may define data as figures. Figures result from the Process of counting or from taking a measurement.

For example:

- When Investigator Counts the Number of patients (***Counting***).
- When Investigator Weighs a patient (***Measurement***)

Variable: It is a characteristic that takes on different values in different persons, places, or things.

For example:

- Heart rate,
- The heights of adult males,
- The pregnancy status of female subjects,
- The Race of patients in clinical study.

Types of Variables

1. Qualitative Variables

Many characteristics are not capable of being measured. Some of them can be ordered or ranked. For example: - Classification of people into Races.

2. Quantitative Variables: It can be measured in the usual sense.

For example:

- The heights of adult males,
- The ages of patients

Types of Quantitative Variables:

A discrete variable is characterized by gaps or interruptions in the values that it can assume.

A continuous variable, can assume any value within a specified relevant interval of values assumed by the variable. For example: Height, weight. No matter how close together the observed heights of two people, we can find another person whose height falls somewhere in between.

Types of Data

1. ***Categorical data:*** values belong to categories

- ✦ Nominal data: there is no natural order to the categories e.g. blood groups
- ✦ Ordinal data: there is natural order e.g. Adverse Events (Mild/ Moderate/Severe/Life Threatening)
- ✦ Binary data: there are only two possible categories e.g. alive/dead

2. ***Numerical data:*** the value is a number (either measured or counted)

- ✦ Continuous data: measurement is on a continuum e.g. height, age, hemoglobin
- ✦ Discrete data: a "count" of events e.g. number of pregnancies

Levels of measurement or Scales of measurement:

In statistics, the term measurement is used more broadly and is more appropriately termed, Scales of measurement. Scales of measurement refer to ways in which variables/numbers are defined and categorized.

Each scale of measurement has certain property which in turn determines the appropriateness for use of certain statistical analyses.

The four scales of measurement are Nominal, Ordinal, Interval, and Ratio.

The relationship of the values that are assigned to the attributes for a variable helps you decide what statistical analysis is appropriate on the values that were assigned.

1. Nominal: The nominal type, sometimes also called the qualitative type, differentiates between items or subjects based only on their categories and other qualitative classifications they belong to. Examples of these classifications include gender, ethnicity, and race.

- Data are coded by a number, name, or letter that is assigned to a category or group Examples :Gender (e.g., male, female)
- When we ask subjects to name their Race, they will respond with words —not numbers—that describe their status such as "Asian," "Black," "White," etc.
- Notice that nominal data do not put subjects in any particular order.
- There is no logical basis for saying that one category such as "Black" is higher or lower than any other.

*2. **Ordinal:*** The ordinal type allows for rank order (1st, 2nd, 3rd, etc.) by which data can be sorted, but still does not allow for relative degree of difference between them.

- Classifies data into categories that can be ordered or ranked, but precise differences between the ranks do not exist.
- Examples: Pain level (e.g., mild, moderate, severe)
- Ordinal values only describe order, not quantity Thus, severe pain is not the same as 2 times mild pain
- Generally it does not make sense to do calculations with data at the ordinal level.
- It is important to note that ranks do not tell us by how much subjects differ.
- The only mathematical operations allowed for nominal and ordinal data are counting of categories e.g., 25 males and 30 females

*3. **Interval:*** Interval level of measurement—ranks data, precise differences between units of measure exist, but there is no meaningful zero.

- If a zero exists, it is an arbitrary point.
- When distance between attributes has meaning, for example, temperature (in Fahrenheit) distance from 30-40 is same as distance from 70-80, Note that ratios don't make any sense -- 80 degrees is not twice as hot as 40 degrees (although the attribute values are).

4. Ratio: Ratio level of measurement—has all the characteristics of the interval level, but a true zero exists. Also, true ratios exist when the same variable is measured on two different members of the population.

Example: Weight of an individual. It makes sense to say that a 80 KG adult weighs twice as much as a 40 KG child.

Descriptive Statistics:

Descriptive statistics are used to describe the distribution of population measurements by providing estimates of central tendency and measures of variability.

- Identifies patterns in the data
- Identifies outliers
- Guides choice of statistical test

Statistical Procedures used to summarize, organize, and simplify data. This Process should be carried out in such a way that reflects overall findings

- Raw data is made more manageable
- Raw data is presented in a logical form
- Patterns can be seen from organized data

Inferential statistics:

Inferential statistics use probability to express the level of certainty about estimates and to test specific hypotheses.

Measures of Central Tendency:

- ***Mean:*** The average of the data, sensitive to outlying data
- ***Median:*** The middle of the data, not sensitive to outlying data
- ***Mode:*** Most commonly occurring value

Measures of variability: Measures of variation give information on the spread or variability of the data values.

- ***Range:*** The spread of the data
- ***IQ range:*** the spread of the data, commonly used for skewed data
- ***Standard deviation:*** a single number which measures how much the observations vary around the mean

- ***Variance:*** Average (approximately) of squared deviations of values from the mean
- ***Coefficient of Variation.***

Shape of a Distribution: Describes how data is distributed, Measures of shape

- ***Symmetrical Data:*** Data that follows normal distribution (mean=median=mode). Report mean & standard deviation & n
- ***Skewed Data:*** Not normally distributed. report Median & IQ Range

DESCRIPTIVE STATISTICS

These are numbers that describe your data and the type of descriptive statistic that should be calculated depends on the type of variable being analyzed: Categorical, Ordinal, or Continuous.

Categorical Variables: Categorical data is data that can take on a discrete number of values or categories with no inherent order to the categories.

Examples of categorical variables are Sex (male or female), Race (Black, White, Asian, and Hispanic), disease or no disease, and yes or no variables.

The types of descriptive statistics that are calculated for categorical variables include frequencies and proportions or percentages in the various categories of the variable.

Ordinal Variables: Ordinal variables are another type of variable where there are a discrete number of values but the values have some inherent order to them. For example, scale variables (strongly disagree, disagree, agree and strongly agree) are ordinal variables.

There is an inherent knowledge that strongly disagree is "worse" than disagree. Several types of descriptive statistics can be calculated for these types of variables including frequencies and proportions or Percentages, Medians, Modes, Inter-quartile range.

Depending on the number of values an ordinal variable can take on, a mean and standard deviation may also be calculated.

Continuous Variables:

Continuous variables are those for which the values can take on an infinite number of values in a given range.

Descriptive statistics that are appropriate for a continuous measure include means, medians, modes, quartiles, variances, standard deviations, coefficients of variation, ranges, minimums, maximums, kurtosis, skewness, inter-quartile ranges, etc..

INFERENTIAL STATISTICS

Hypothesis: A hypothesis is a proposed explanation for a phenomenon.

Null Hypothesis: the null hypothesis refers to a general statement or default position that there is no relationship between two measured phenomena.

Reject Null Hypothesis: (Rejecting or disproving the null hypothesis) – concluding that there are grounds for believing that there is a relationship between two phenomena.

P-Value: is the probability of obtaining a test statistic result at least as extreme as the one that was actually observed, assuming that the null hypothesis is true. A Statistician will often "reject the null hypothesis" when the p-value turns out to be less than a predetermined significance level, often 0.05 or 0.01.

Statistical significance is the low probability that an observed effect would have occurred due to chance. It is an integral part of statistical hypothesis testing where it helps investigators to decide if a null hypothesis can be rejected.

Alpha Error: A type I error, also known as an error of the first kind, occurs when the null hypothesis (H0) is true, but is rejected.

Beta Error: A type II error, also known as an error of the second kind, occurs when the null hypothesis is false, but erroneously fails to be rejected.

	Null hypothesis (H0) is true	Null hypothesis (H0) is false
Reject null hypothesis	Type I error False positive	Correct outcome True positive
Fail to reject null hypothesis	Correct outcome True negative	Type II error False negative

Types of Clinical Studies

1) Observational Studies

- ***Cohort:*** Follow patients with a risk factor to see incidence of disease (prospective).
- ***Cross-sectional:*** Assess risk factor and disease simultaneously (longitudinal).
- ***Case-control:*** Identify patients with and without a disease, and compare histories of treatments and risk factors (retrospective).

2) Experimental Studies

- Randomized
- Controlled
- Blinded
- Crossover
- Open-label

Randomized, Controlled, Double-blind:

- Most common type
- Randomly assigned to treatment group
- Comparison group (Control)
- Patient, Site personnel are blinded to treatment

Elements of a GOOD Study:

- Objective
- Treatment/risk factor and outcome variables
- Hypothesis
- Population
- Inclusion/exclusion criteria
- Time frame

Research Questions:

- ***Comparison of treatments:*** Does Treatment A reduce blood pressure more effectively than Treatment B?
- ***Evaluating one treatment:*** Does Treatment A reduce the risk of MI?

- ***Retrospective:*** Is chronic caffeine consumption associated with hypertension?
- ***Prospective:*** What is the incidence of lung cancer among tobacco users?

Does Treatment A reduce blood pressure more effectively than Treatment B?

- ***Objective:*** To determine which drug reduces blood pressure more effectively.
- ***Treatment:*** Treatment A (dose 10mg/day) or Treatment B (dose 10mg/day).
- ***Outcome:*** Blood pressure.
- ***Hypothesis:*** Treatment A will result in lower SBP than Treatment B.
- ***Time frame:*** 3 months of treatment.
- ***Population:*** Hypertensive patients.
- ***Criteria:*** Hypertension, age 55+, no previous use of Treatments A or B

Evaluating One Treatment:

Does Treatment A reduce the risk of MI?

- ***Objective:*** To determine whether Treatment A reduces the incidence of second MI.
- ***Treatment:*** Treatment A (dose 10mg /day).
- ***Outcome:*** Myocardial Infarction.
- ***Hypothesis:*** Treatment A will result in lower rate of MI compared to placebo.
- ***Time frame:*** 5 years.
- ***Population:*** Patients at Present with history of MI.
- ***Criteria:*** Previous MI, no previous use of Treatment A, no diabetes.

Selection of an appropriate statistical test

Prior to selecting a Statistical Test we need ask the following questions,

- ✦ Type of the Data (N,O,I,R)
- ✦ What we want to Analyze? (Association, Difference, Prediction etc)
- ✦ How many Variables are there to Analyze?
- ✦ What Statistics are required? (Descriptive, Inferential)

1. Description of one group:

- ✦ ***Nominal*** → Proportion → Proc Freq
- ✦ ***Ordinal, R/I (Not Normally Distributed)*** → Median, IQ range →Proc Univariate, Means
- ✦ ***R/I(Normally Distributed)*** → Mean, SD →Proc Univariate, Proc Means

2. Comparison of one group to a Hypothetical Value:

- ✦ ***Nominal*** → Chi square, Binomial → Proc Freq
- ✦ ***Ordinal, R/I (NND)*** → Wilcoxon Signed Rank Test →Proc Univariate
- ✦ ***R/I(ND)*** → One Sample Ttest, Z test →Proc Univariate, Proc Ttest

3. Comparison of Two Groups (Paired Groups):

- ✦ ***Nominal*** → Mc Nemars Test → Proc Freq
- ✦ ***Ordinal, R/I (NND)***→Wilcoxon T (Matched Pair)Test →Proc Npar1way
- ✦ ***R/I (ND)*** → Paired Ttest →Proc Ttest

4. Comparison of Two Groups (Unpaired Groups):

- ✦ ***Nominal*** → Fishers Exact, Chi square(n>30) →Proc Freq
- ✦ ***Ordinal, R/I (NND)*** → Wilcoxon Rank Sum Test, →Mann Whitney U Test →Proc Npar1way
- ✦ ***R/I (ND)*** → Unpaired Ttest →Proc Ttest

5. Comparison of Three or more Groups (Matched Groups):

- ***Nominal*** → Cochran Q → Proc Freq
- ***Ordinal, R/I (NND)*** → Friedman Test →
- ***R/I (ND)*** → Repeated Measures Anova →Proc Anova, Proc GLM

6. Comparison of Three or more Groups (Unmatched Groups):

- ***Nominal*** → Chi square → Proc Freq
- ***Ordinal, R/I (NND)*** → Kruskal Wallis Test →Proc Npar1way
- ***R/I (ND)*** → One way Anova →Proc Anova

7. Measures of Association between Two variables:

- ***Nominal*** → Contingency Co-efficient → Proc Freq
- ***Ordinal, R/I (NND)*** → Spearman Correlation →Proc Corr
- ***R/I (ND)*** → Pearson Correlation →Proc Corr

8. Prediction: From another measured Variable:

- ***Nominal*** → Simple Logistic Regression → Proc Logistic
- ***Ordinal, R/I (NND)*** → Non Parametric Regression → Proc GAM
- ***R/I (ND)*** → Simple Linear Regression →Proc Reg

Proc Freq (FREQ Procedure)

The FREQ Procedure produces one-way to n-way frequency and cross tabulation (contingency) tables. For two-way tables, PROC FREQ computes tests and measures of association. For n-way tables, PROC FREQ does stratified analysis, computing statistics within, as well as across, strata. Frequencies and statistics can also be output to SAS data sets.

Syntax of Proc Freq:

```
Proc FREQ < Options >;
TABLES Requests < / Options >;
BY Variables;
WEIGHT Variable < / Option >;
TEST Options;
EXACT Statistic-Options < / computation-options >;
OUTPUT < OUT=SAS-data-set > Options;
RUN;
```

Let us begin by asking for frequencies (one-way) on each of the variables of interest SEX and AGE (Age variable is continuous, we cannot use Proc Freq), we can use Proc Freq on Agegrp Variable (Age Variable is Grouped).

To obtain One-Way Freq on Single variable

```
PROC FREQ Data=YLP.Dmads;
Tables Sex;
Run;
```

By executing the above Proc step we obtained

- Frequency
- Percent
- Cumulative Frequency
- Cumulative Percent on SEX variable

If we want to obtain One-Way Freq on Multiple Variables we use both the variables in Tables statement separated by space.

- To obtain this we use the TABLES statement, we list both variables separated by a space.

```
Proc Freq Data= YLP.Dmads;
Tables Sex Agegrp;
Run;
```

If we need to perform analysis on only those patients who are male, we use a WHERE statement

Proc Freq Data= YLP.Dmads;

Tables Trtcd;

*Where Sex=2; *provided Males are coded as 2;*

Run;

By default Proc freq will not consider the missing values into analysis, if we want to analyze missing values we need to use an option 'Missing'.

Proc Freq Data= YLP.Dmads;

Tables Sex/ Missing;

Run;

As per the Mock shell (Look at the Table2 in Mock shells), we require Gender and Agegrp statistics against Treatment, to obtain these ***Cross Tabular Freq***, we use Tables statement in which the variables are ***separated by Asterisk***.

Proc Freq Data= YLP.Dmads;

*Tables Sex*Trtcd;*

*Tables Agegrp*Trtcd;*

Run;

By executing the above Proc step we obtained

- ✦ Frequency
- ✦ Percent
- ✦ Row Percent
- ✦ Column Percent by default

To make the report more understandable we apply Formats for the Frequency report

Creating Format

Proc Format;

Value Sexfmt 1='Female' 2='Male';

Value Trtfmt 1='Placebo'

2='TD1mg'

3='TD3mg'

4='TD6mg';

Run;

Once we have our format created, we need to apply the format with a FORMAT statement in PROC FREQ.

To create cross tabular freq report with formats:

Proc Freq Data= YLP.Dmads;

Format Sex Sexfmt. Trtcd trtfmt.;

*Tables Sex*Trtcd;*

Run;

PROC FREQ will by default add several unwanted statistics to the table, when we define two dimensions, if we want to suppress Row pct, Col pct and Overall pct, We can add the ***NOROW NOCOL, and NOPERCENT options.***

Proc Freq Data= YLP.Dmads;

Format Sex Sexfmt. Trtcd Trtfmt.;

*Tables Sex*Trtcd /* ***Norow Nocol Nopercent****;*

Run;

We can even add a LABEL statement to further describe the variables in our report.

Proc Freq Data= YLP.Dmads;

Tables Sex Trtcd/ norow nocol nopercent;*

LABEL Trtcd = 'Trt assigned to Patient' Sex='Sex of Patient';

Run;

Creating a dataset with the Statistics

Proc Freq Data=YLP.Dmads;

*Tables Sex*Trtcd /* ***Out=freqds;***

Run;

- ***Out= option*** is to create a new dataset, by default, we get only Freq, Percent in new dataset.
- ***Outpct option*** is to obtain Rowpct and Colpct in new dataset.
- To suppress the listing (.lst) report we use ***Noprint Option***;

Proc Freq Data=YLP.Dmads ***Noprint;***

*Tables Sex*Trtcd/ Out=freqds* ***Outpct;***

Run;

CHI-Square Test

Chi-Square: A test of significance used with cross tabulations of nominal/ordinal level data. The chi-square test is useful for detection of a general association between treatment and categorical response (in either the nominal or ordinal scale), but it cannot identify a particular relationship.

The chi-square test is used to ***compare two independent binomial proportions***, p1 and p2.

In the analysis of clinical data, the binomial proportion typically represents:

- Response rate,
- Cure rate,
- Survival rate,
- Abnormality rate,
- 'Event' rate

Often, you want to compare such 'Response' rates between treated group and control group.

The chi-square test is an approximate test, which may be used when the normal approximation to the binomial distribution is valid. Chi-square statistic can be obtained by using ***CHISQ Option***.

Chi-Square compares the observed frequencies (from the data in your sample) to expected frequencies.

Expected frequencies: These are the frequencies we would expect if the null hypothesis were true

```
Data Trial;
Input TRT $ AE $ CNT @@;
Datalines;
Active YES 29 Active NO 21
Control YES 16 Control NO 34
;
Run;

Proc Freq Data= Trial;
Tables TRT*AE / CHISQ NOPERCENT NOCOL;
Weight CNT;
Run;

Proc Freq Data = Trial;
Tables TRT*AE / Chisq;
Weight CNT;
Output Out=Chs_sta Chisq;
Run;
```

- By executing the above step we created a dataset named Chs_sta in which we can observe many variables with p – values like Chi Square (P_PCHI) , Fisher's Exact (XP2_FISH), Mantel-Heanszel (P_MHCHI) etc.,

Since the variables TRT and AE in the above dataset are binomial, independent variables we consider Chi Square test under the assumption that normal approximation to the binomial distribution is valid.

```
To pick the required p-value (Chi-Square);
Data Chstat;
Set Chs_sta (Keep=P_pchi);
Run;
```

EXAMPLES OF CATEGORICAL DATA:

Nominal:

- **Treatment** -- *Active, Control (Binomial)*
- **Response** -- *Yes, No (Binomial)*
- **Race** -- *Caucasian, Black, Hispanic (Nominal)*
- **Lesion Site** -- *Leg, Back, Arm, Face, Chest (Nominal)*
- **Treatment** -- *Active, Placebo, Reference (Nominal)*

Ordinal:

- **Improvement**-- *Worse, None, Some, Marked, Cured*
- **Severity** -- *None, Mild, Moderate, Severe*
- **Dosage** -- *1 mg, 3mg, 6mg*

Using Weight Statement:

Let us assume that, we introduced an Intervention and surveyed the ***SAME 100 patients*** after the Intervention. We want to know if there has been a significant change or shift in the patient's original opinion (Yes or No) on some parameter.

```
Data Trial;
Input Pre $ Post $ Count;
Datalines;
Yes Yes 30
Yes No 10
No Yes 40
No No 20
;
Run;
```

- 30 patients answered Yes initially and at follow-up.
- 10 patients answered Yes initially and then No at follow-up.
- 40 patients answered No initially and then Yes at follow-up.
- 20 patients answer No initially and then No at follow-up.

In the above dataset we have three variables, in that Two Variables (Pre and Post) are Categorical and Binomial. So since we are ***analyzing***

two binomial variables we tend to go with CHISQ test, but we cannot use the CHISQ option with PROC FREQ here, because these variables ***are not independent groups***. They are in fact the same 100 patients who we surveyed initially and then after 10 weeks. The SAS System has an option in Proc Freq to handle this type of analysis. It is the ***AGREE option***.

```
PROC Freq Data=Trial;
TABLES Pre*Post / AGREE;
WEIGHT Count;
RUN;
```

We have replaced the CHISQ option with the AGREE option since we are working with data that is ***not independent*** (actually called paired data). The WEIGHT statement is used since without it SAS would report that we only had 4 observations instead of 100 observations.

Fisher's Exact Test:

Fisher's exact test is an alternative to the chi-square test for comparing two independent binomial proportions, p1 and p2. This method is based on computing exact probabilities of observing a given result or a more extreme result, when the hypothesis of equal proportions is true.

Fisher's exact test is useful when the normal approximation to the binomial might not be applicable, such as in the case of small cell sizes or extreme proportions.

```
Data Test;
Input Trt Resp $ Cnt @@;
Datalines;
1 YES 2 1 NO 33
2 YES 5 2 NO 15
;
Run;
```

Fisher's exact test is considered a non-parametric test because it does not rely on any distributional assumptions. Fisher's Exact statistic can be obtained by using ***EXACT Option***

```
Proc Freq Data = Test;
Tables Trt*Resp / Fisher Nopercent Nocol;
Weight Cnt;
Output out=fqex Exact;
Run;
```

Keep only XP2_FISH variable for Exact P-value.

Mantel-Heanszel Chi-Square Test

```
Data Trial;
Input Sex $ Trt $ Response $ Count @@;
Datalines;
Female test none 6 female test some 5
Female test marked 16 female placebo none 19
Female placebo some 7 female placebo marked 6
Male test none 7 male test some 2
Male test marked 5 male placebo none 10
Male placebo some 0 male placebo marked 1
;
Run;
```

In the above dataset we can observe that ***Trt*** variable have two values ***(Binomial)*** where as ***Response*** variables are an ***Ordinal Variable*** (None, Some, Marked). In this situation we consider Mantel-Heanszel Chi-Square Test.

```
Proc Freq Data=Trial;
Weight count;
Tables Trt*Response / Chisq ;
Run;
```

Keep only P_MHCHI Variable for Mantel-Heanszel P-value.

Cochran-Mantel-Heanszel Chi-Square Test (CMH Test)

If we want to know the output of treat*response by each Gender in our study, we can add another dimension to our TABLES statement to accomplish this task. With a two-way table the first dimension is the ROW and the second dimension is the COLUMN. If we have a three-way Crosstab then the first dimension is the STRATA, the second dimension is the ROW and the third dimension is the COLUMN.

```
Proc Freq Data=Trial;
Weight Count;
Tables Sex*Trt*Response / CMH Nocol Nopercent;
Run;
```

Proc Means (MEANS Procedure)

The MEANS Procedure provides data summarization tools to compute descriptive statistics, Hypothesis Testing across all observations and within groups of observations.

Syntax of Proc Means:

```
PROC MEANS Options;
BY variable(s);
CLASS variable(s);
VAR variable(s);
WEIGHT variable;
FREQ variable;
TYPES request(s);
WAYS list;
OUTPUT ...;
Run;
```

The PROC MEANS statement is the only required statement for the MEANS Procedure. If you specify the following statements, Proc Means produces five basic stats (N, Min, Max, Mean, SD) for each numeric variable in the last created dataset.

Proc Means;

Run;

If we want to know the Average ***Age*** (Mean) of the patients, we can use Proc means in the following way with ***VAR Statement***. In Var Statement we should give the analysis variable.

Proc Means Data=YLP. Dmads Mean;

Var Ageyr;

Run;

Using the CLASS Statement:

The CLASS statement can be used to create subgroups. Unlike the BY statement the data do not have to be sorted prior to its use. Like in most other Procedures that utilize the CLASS statement, there can be one or more classification variables.

If we want to know what are the mean age of the Men and the mean age of the Women, we can add a CLASS statement to our program.

Proc Means Data= YLP. Dmads Mean;

Var Ageyr;

Class Sex;

Run;

Another way to calculate the mean age of men and the mean age of women is to use a BY statement instead of a CLASS statement. The only caveat is that whenever you use a BY statement, the SAS dataset must be sorted.

While we have concisely produced the above table without sorting the data and using the CLASS statement we could still do more to present it aesthetically pleasing to the eye. So let's decrease the decimal places to 2 (Two) by using ***Maxdec=*** Option and Format the Sex variable with Format Statement.

```
Proc Format;
Value Sexfmt 1='F:Female' 2='M:Male';
Run;

Proc Means Data=YLP. Dmads Maxdec=2;
Class Sex;
Var Ageyr;
Format Sex Sexfmt.;
Run;
```

Suppose that we want to see the MEAN, MEDIAN and the 90% Confidence Limits of the Mean. Whenever we want anything other than the default statistics we have to explicitly ask for them.

```
Proc Means Data=YLP.Dmads Mean Median CLM  ALPHA= 0.10
Maxdec=2;
Class Sex;
Var Ageyr;
Run;
```

- ***ALPHA*** in the above Program specifies the Probability of committing Type 1 Error (Rejecting the True Null Hypothesis).
- Type 2 Error (Beta Error) Fail to reject the False Null Hypothesis

Suppose that we wanted to store the Proc Means generated analyses in a SAS data set instead of placing them in the Output Window. We can do this by including an ***OUTPUT Statement*** as part of the Proc Means task, which will control what variables and observations are placed in to the data set.

```
Proc Means Data=YLP.Dmads Noprint;
Class Sex;
Var Ageyr;
Output out=avgds;
Run;
```

Output out=Dsname n=number mean=average std=std_deviation; This allows you to name more than one statistic on the OUTPUT statement.

By executing the above program we created a dataset with three new variables (Automatic).

- _TYPE_
- _STAT_
- _FREQ_

Understanding _TYPE_ Automatic variable:

The _TYPE_ variable in the output data set helps us track the level of summarization, and can be used to distinguish the sets of statistics. Notice in the previous example that _TYPE_ changes for each level of summarization.

- _TYPE_ = 0 Summarize across all classification variables
- _TYPE_ = 1 Summarize as if the right most classification variable (SEX) was the only one
- _TYPE_ = 2 Summarize as if the next to the right most classification variable (SEX) was the only one
- _TYPE_ = 3 Interaction of the two classification variables.

```
Proc Means Data=YLP.Dmads Noprint;
Var Ageyr;
Output out=avgds1;
Run;

Proc Means Data=YLP. Dmads Noprint;
Class Sex;
Var Ageyr;
Output out=avgds2;
Run;

Proc Means Data=YLP. Dmads Noprint;
Class Trt Sex;
Var Ageyr;
Output out=avgds3;
Run;
```

Compare three datasets Avgds 1, 2, 3 to understand how _Type_ works.

Automatic Naming of Summary Variables: When you do not need to control the naming of the new summary variables, the ***AUTONAME and AUTOLABEL options*** can be used on the OUTPUT statement.

```
Proc Means Data=YLP. Dmads Noprint;
Class Trt;
Var Ageyr;
Output out=avgds N = Mean= Std = / Autoname;
Run;
```

Proc Univariate (UNIVARIATE Procedure)

This is a Procedure used primarily for examining the distribution of data, including an assessment of normality and discovery of outliers.

- ✦ It provides a variety of descriptive measures, high-resolution graphical displays, and statistical methods, which can be used to summarize, visualize, analyze, and model the statistical distributions of numeric variables.

Statements used in PROC UNIVARIATE:

```
PROC UNIVARIATE < options > ;
CLASS variable(s);
VAR variable(s);
BY variable(s);
ID variable(s ;
OUTPUT < OUT=SAS-data-set > < percentile-options >;
WEIGHT variable;
Run;
```

PROC UNIVARIATE will produce for each numeric variable in the last created dataset:

- ✦ ***Moments*** - N, Mean, Standard Deviation, Uncorrected Sum of Squares, Coefficient of Variation, Sum of Weights, Sum of Observations, Variance, Kurtosis, Corrected Sum of Squares and Standard Error of the Mean etc.

- ***Basic Statistical Measures:*** - Mean, Median, Mode, Standard Deviation, Variance, Range and Inter quartile Range
- ***Tests for Location*** Mu0=0 - Student's t, Sign and Signed Rand tests with their associated p-values
- ***Quantiles*** - 0%(Min), 1%, 5%, 10%, 25%(Q1), 50%(Median), 75%(Q3), 90%, 95%, 99% and 100%(Max)
- ***Extreme Observations*** - the five lowest and the five highest values

Proc Univariate Data= YLP.Dmads;

Class Sex;

Var Ageyr;

Run;

- By executing the above Procedure we created descriptive statistics on Ageyr variable based on their sex.

There are some common options used in the Proc Univariate statement are DATA=, NORMAL, FREQ, PLOT.

These options are explained as follows:

- The DATA= option specifies which SAS Dataset to use in the PROC
- The ***NORMAL option*** indicates a request for several tests of normality of variable(s)
- The ***Freq option*** produces a frequency table of the variable(s)
- The ***Plot option*** produces stem-and-leaf, box - whisker plots etc

If we want to look at the variable AGE grouped by the SEX variable, we can do this by using a CLASS statement. The dataset does not have to be sorted.

Proc Univariate Data= YLP. Dmads;

Class Sex;

Var Ageyr;

Run;

The above step will give us two reports. One will be all the moments, basic statistical measures, tests for location, quantiles and extreme observations for females. The other report will be the same five reports for the males.

```
Proc Univariate Data=YLP.CFB NORMAL;
Var baseline vsrn change;
Run;
```

To test for normality you must add the keyword normal (or normal test) to the Proc Univariate statement. Proc Univariate displays two statistics in the Tests for Normality section. These are W and D SAS uses the ***Shapiro-Wilk test*** when the sample size is below 2000 and the ***Kolmogorov-Smirnov test*** for sample size above 2000.

Let us assume that the following patients are in weight reduction treatment for 2 months, and the data looks like this

```
Data Wtred;
Input Patid Chg_val @@;
Datalines;
101 -3 102 0 103 -4 104 -7 106 -5
110 -8 112 -6 113 -9 115 -6 120 -4
;
Run;
```

To obtain descriptive as well as inferential stats on single continuous variable

```
Proc Univariate Data=Wtred NORMAL;
Var chg_val;
Run;
```

Comparing the Test drug with Standard drug (Which reduces 3 kg)

```
Proc Univariate Data=Wtred normal mu0= -3;
Var chg_val;
Run;
```

Based on the Normality of the continuous variable, we pick proper statistical test

- Normal Distribution → ***Students T Test***
- Not Normal Distribution → Sign Test (Skewed Distribution)
Signed Rank test (Symmetric Distribution)

Proc Univariate in Data Cleaning:

- Timely and strategic cleaning of data is crucial for the success of the analysis of a clinical trial.
- Data quality is essential for the trustworthiness of the final analysis that determines if a drug is efficacious or safe, and thus worthy of regulatory approval.
- With the introduction of Electronic Data Capture, expectations are that these timelines should fall further.
- However, there still remains a risk that data may not be quite what it was expected to be. This may be attributable to unforeseen bias emerging at sites, and so it is useful to establish this as early as possible in the trial to determine if the expected statistical model was wrong.
- When outliers become extreme observations at either the left or the right it could alter the assumptions made by the statistician at study set-up about the behavior of the recruited population - which could jeopardize the proof of the trial.
- The extreme observations are the ones of interest and deserve our attention as being more than just the normal outliers at the end of the bell-curve. These are the ones that skew the distribution into the F-shape.
- UNIVARIATE by default lists the top 5 and bottom 5 observations (identified by the VAR statement) ranked in term of their value.
- The numbers to be displayed can be controlled by the ***NEXTROBS option*** of UNIVARIATE.

```
ODS Select ExtremeObs;
Proc Univariate Data=YLP.Labs NEXTROBS=10;
Class lbtest;
Id patid;
Var Lbrn;
Run;
```

As per mock shell (Check Table2 in Mock shells) we require to present N, Mean, Std, Median, Min, Max statistics.

```
Proc Univariate data = YLP.Dmads Noprint;
By Trt;
Var Ageyr;
Output out = ageds n = _n median= _median mean = _mean std = _std
min = _min max = _max;
Run;

Data agefin;
Set ageds;
Format n mean std min max $14.;
Drop _n _mean _std _min _max;
N = put(_n,3.);
Mean = put(_mean,5.1);
Std = put(_std,6.2);
Median=put(_median,5.1);
Min = put(_min,5.1);
Max = put(_max,5.1);
Run;
```

ODS (Output Delivery System)

SAS programmers in the Clinical industry needs to present the summary tables and listings as part of electronic submissions (eSub) as per FDA guidelines.

Proc steps create Output Objects, by default going to output window (.Lst report). ODS output is created from the Procedure output, a table definition, a style definition, and a destination.

- ***Procedure Output:*** This is the text and numbers that make up your results.
- ***Table Definition:*** Each Procedure has a table definition that tells it how to arrange, display, and label the results.
- ***Style Definition:*** This defines the appearance of the output, and includes color schemes, fonts, borders, and sizes.
- ***Output Destination:*** Output can be sent to an HTML file, a PDF file, a RTF document, or many other destinations.

The output object is the foundation of ODS. Almost every SAS Procedure uses output objects. There are two types of output objects created by ODS:

- Tabular output objects
- Graphical output objects.

No matter which type of output object your Procedure creates, you can discover useful information about the object with the ODS TRACE statement. If you use the ODS TRACE statement, you can see in the SAS log that each output object has other attributes in addition to the Name attribute.

The five most common attributes are:

1. Name
2. Label
3. Template
4. Path
5. Label Path.

If we can track the output object and specify the destination, we can create the reports in user defined destinations.

Different Destinations:

- Listing (.LST) – Default (Output Window)
- Output -- Output Dataset
- Html(.HTML) -- Hyper Text Markup Language(Web Sharing)

- Word Doc (.RTF) -- Rich Text Format
- PDF (.PDF) -- Portable Document Format

The Reporting Output section in SAP (Statistical Analysis Plan), would mention the reports need to be created and their extensions (RTF, .PDF etc)

```
Data Test;
Input Wt_Chg @@;
Datalines;
2 9 7 4 3 6 4 8 5 2
;
Run;

Proc Univariate Data=Test;
Var Wt_Chg;
Run;
```

By executing the above Procedure we created, by default .lst report in output window with five sections as follows:

- Moments
- Basic Statistical Measures
- Tests For Location
- Quantiles
- Extreme Observations

Output producing Procedures often create multiple pieces or tables of information. In order to discriminate between the various pieces of information, it is advantageous to know the names assigned to each piece of information. The ability to display the names of individual pieces of information generated on output is referred to as TRACING.

The ***ODS statement syntax:*** *ODS trace ON / Listing;*

Causes the SAS System to turn the trace feature on and print results to the SAS Listing destination.

```
ODS Trace ON / Listing;
Proc univariate data=Test;
Run;
```

ODS Trace Off;

The trace record displays information about the data component, the table definition, and the output object. For example, the trace record displays the following output objects to the SAS Listing destination:

1) Moments 2) BasicMeasures 3) TestForLocation 4) Quantiles and 5) ExtremeObs.

Note that for each output object, the name, label, template, and path is displayed.

Once you know the individual names of each output object (from the trace), you can then select the desired object for reporting purposes by using ***ODS Select Statement***.

The syntax is: ODS SELECT Output-Component-Name;

Where output-component-name is the name of the desired output object.

To select just the output object Moments from the Univariate Procedure, the following syntax is specified:

ODS Select Moments;

Proc univariate data=Test;

Run;

Occasionally, output results are needed in a SAS data set rather than in printed form such as the Listing destination. Re-directing SAS Procedure output to a data set is relatively simple with ODS by using ***ODS Output Statement***.

The syntax is: ODS Output output-table-name = user-defined-table-name;

Where output-table-name is the name of the desired output table (component) containing the information you want written to a data set, such as Moments in the UNIVARIATE Procedure. User-defined-table-name is the name you supply for the newly created data set.

It can be defined as either a temporary or permanent data set. Once an object is selected, specify the object in the ODS OUTPUT statement.

Creating Rich Text Format (RTF) with ODS:

A document using a SAS Mono space 8 pt. font, the readability of the table is at the limit of acceptability. If we had longer treatment group labels, longer parameter names or additional groups to present it would be difficult to display the table without compromising readability. Rich text format (RTF) is text consisting of formatting attributes codes, such as boldface, italics, underline, etc.

The syntax to create RTF output is:

ODS RTF FILE = 'user-specified-file-name';

Where user-specified-file-name references complete and fully-qualified output location for the creation and storage of the RTF file, data, and codes. For example, the following code creates an RTF file using the Univariate Procedure output.

ODS RTF FILE='E:\Ods reports\test.rtf';

Proc univariate data=Test;

Run;

ODS RTF Close;

ADVANTAGES OF ODS RTF:

The appearance of tables with relatively large quantities of data is enhanced through the use of more legible proportional fonts, use of color, and division of tables by lines. Proportional fonts and lines dividing the table into cells allow data to be displayed in a tighter space without compromising readability.

The Listing destination is open by default at SAS invocation, while the other destinations are closed. If nothing is done to suppress output to the Listing destination, your SAS programs automatically produce Listing output, just as they always have in the SAS System. If you need to suppress printed output from being sent to the Listing destination before the execution of a Procedure step, the following ODS statement would be issued: ***ODS Listing Close.***

ODS Listing Close;

Proc univariate data=Test;

Run;

ODS Listing;

By closing the Listing destination before the Procedure code, the SAS System is actually suppressing output to that destination until it is reopened. The preceding example shows that at the end of the Procedure step, the Listing destination is reopened by specifying ODS Listing, so output from subsequent steps can be sent to the Listing destination.

To provide greater capabilities when working with custom output created in the DATA step, ODS is integrated into the DATA step.

Two new options are necessary to take advantage of ODS:

- ✦ The ODS option in the FILE statement and
- ✦ The _ODS_ option in the PUT statement.

These two options are used to direct the results of a DATA step to ODS. For example, the following code directs output from a DATA step through the RTF format engine to create a RTF file.

ODS RTF FILE='E:\Ods reports\DSrep.rtf';

Data NULL;

Set Test;

File print ODS;

Put _ODS_;

Run;

ODS RTF Close;

ADDING STYLE TO YOUR REPORTS:

If you want to change the way the reports as per client requirements SAS provides many pre-packaged styles that you can use for your reports. However, destinations that are usually used for printing looks better without background colors.

Output Delivery System (ODS), provides the ability to both greatly enhance the appearance of tabular output and to meet the FDA's guidelines.

FDA Electronic Submission Guidelines:

- ✦ Font size as close to 12 as possible
- ✦ Paper size 8.5 x 11 inches
- ✦ Margins at least 1 inch on all sides
- ✦ Use only True Type or Adobe Type 1 fonts
- ✦ Limit the number of fonts in each document
- ✦ Embed all fonts in the PDF file

Based upon the unofficial rule, when producing listings and tables, we are limited to a SAS output file line size of about 140characters maximum. These files can then be converted into documents with fonts of 8 point. This is the outer limit of acceptability, and in many cases can impede our ability to present the data as we like.

Locate Existing Styles:

There are different styles provided with SAS. They are located in the SASHELP.TMPLMST template store.

A template store is a specially formatted file that is created by PROC TEMPLATE. The styles are stored in the Styles folder of the SASHELP.TMPLMST template store.

Proc Template;

List styles;

Run;

Although the styles provided by SAS are nice, if none of those styles is exactly matches your want. Fortunately, you can define your own; unfortunately, this can be a rather daunting task.

In-Line Formatting:

In-line formatting is a powerful tool to let you insert custom formatting anywhere there is text in your ODS output. This technique does not work for Listing Output; in fact it will make a mess of your listing output. But for HTML, RTF, and PDF, it is very powerful.

The first step is to turn on in-line formatting. This is done by specifying a special character to be used to identify in-line formatting sequences.

- This needs to be a character that won't be needed anywhere else in the output.
- One popular character to use is the caret ('^'), but the choice is up to you.
- The syntax for identifying the character is: ***ODS ESCAPECHAR='^';***

The next step is to find a way to apply the formatting to the appropriate text. In this example, we will add the footnotes to selected row headings by adding the formatting characters to the

PROC FORMAT labels for each row. To indicate a superscript, the escape character is followed by a special command in brackets. For a superscript, the command is the keyword, super, followed by a space, followed by the text to superscript.

Proc Format;

value txft 1='Control'

2='Low Dose^{super 1}'

3='High Dose^{super 2}';

Run;

However, the footnotes look a little odd because they are so much bigger than the table text. To fix this, we can add just the font size used in the footnotes via another in-line formatting command. The style command uses a capital 'S' followed by an equal sign and then brackets containing a style attribute.

Footnote "^S={font_size=2}^{Placebo}2 ml/kg.";

Footnote2 "^S={font_size=2}^{Active}5 ml/kg";

Proc Ttest (TTEST Procedure)

Parametric data are analyzed using statistical techniques identified as Parametric Statistics. As a rule, there are more statistical technique options for the analysis of parametric data and parametric statistics are considered more powerful than non-parametric.

Parametric means that it meets certain requirements with respect to parameters of the population (for example, the data will be normal - the distribution parallels the normal or bell curve). In addition, it means that numbers can be added, subtracted, multiplied, and divided.

There are different Ttest based on No. of variables to analyze

- ✦ One Sample Ttest (1 Var), Paired Sample Ttest (Same Var Collected Two times)
- ✦ Two Sample Ttest

One- Sample Ttest:

- ✦ We use this test to compare a sample mean to a given value
- ✦ We use Ttest when we have the confirmation that the data follows assumptions on distribution.

```
Data Trial;
Input patid chg_val @@;
Datalines;
101 3 102 0 103 4 104 7 106 5
110 8 112 6 113 9 115 4 120 4
;
Run;
```

Obtaining inferential statistics and comparing the P-Value

```
Proc Ttest Data=Trial;
Var chg_val;
Run;
```

- By submitting the above program we got the results in the output window, we need to consider Pr>|t| value as P-value.
- Since the obtained P-value is 0.0002 we can ***reject the null hypothesis*** stating that there is significant difference between compared groups (Test Drug Vs No Trt).
- If the client specifies the standard Trt value as 4, and we are supposed to compare our mean change with standard value.

If we want to create a dataset with the p-value we use ODS facility

```
ODS Trace On;
Proc Ttest Data=Trial;
Var chg_val;
ODS Output ttests = pval;
Run;
ODS Trace Off;
Data Pvalue (keep = Probt); /*Probt is the variable name, Pr>|t| is Label*/
Set pval;
Run;
```

The paired-difference t-test is a parametric test for comparing paired groups.

The two assumptions for the paired-difference t-test are the following:

- Each pair of measurements is independent of other pairs of measurements
- Differences are from a normal distribution

```
DATA pairtt;
Input Patid Bl_val Pt_val @@;
Datalines;
101 83 80 102 90 90
103 74 70 104 84 77
106 74 72 110 89 80
112 86 85 113 99 92
115 84 80
;
Run;
```

In the above Dataset, we have two Variables Bl_Val and Pt_Val of the same measurement collected at two different time points

Comparing the change value with Standard Drug;

```
Proc Ttest Data=pairtt h0=3;
Paired bl_val*pt_val;
Run;
```

- The PAIRED statement identifies the two variables that contain the original pairs of information.
- In the PAIRED statement, an asterisk separates the two variables. This special use of the asterisk is not interpreted as multiply. Instead, the asterisk tells the Procedure to subtract the second variable from the first variable.

Two Sample Ttest

The two-sample Ttest is a parametric test for comparing two independent groups.

The three assumptions for the two-sample Ttest are the following:

- Observations are independent
- Observations in each group are a random sample from a population with a normal distribution
- Variances for the two independent groups are equal

```
DATA Test;
Input Patid Trt $ Chg_val @@;
Datalines;
101 a 6 102 p 1 103 a 7 104 a 3
105 p 0 106 a 2 107 p 4 108 a 8
109 p 0 110 a 11 111 a 6 112 p 2
;
Run;
```

To check the Variances equality:

H0: MuA=MuB (the Variance between two groups are equal)

```
Proc Ttest data=Test ;
Class Trt;
Var Chg_val;
Run;
```

- By executing the above Procedure and considering the P_value i.e. Pr> F. Since the obtained P-Value is 0.2719 we fail to reject null hypothesis and conclude that there is no much evidence to prove that there is significant difference between variances
- Here the continuous variable is normally distributed and the categorical variable having two responses

```
ODS Output ttests=pval;
Proc Ttest Data=Test;
Class Trt; *categorical data;
Var chg_val; *analysis variable;
Run;
```

ODS Output Close;

In the output dataset we need to consider Probt variable as the P-value

Proc Npar1way (NPAR1WAY Procedure)

PROC NPAR1WAY (Nonparametric 1-way Analysis of variance) is a Non parametric method, the term "Non-Parametric" is not meant to imply that the number and nature of the parameters is flexible and not fixed in advance and they do not assume an underlying parametric distribution such as normal for the data. Non-parametric models are therefore also called "distribution free". Non Parametric methods are particularly useful when data consist of ranks (and not values) of random variables.

The NPAR1WAY Procedure computes exact p-values for the simple linear rank statistics based on ***Wilcoxon scores***, Median scores, Van Der Waerden scores, and Savage scores.

For the two-sample case, the simple linear rank statistics listed above correspond to the ***Wilcoxon-Mann-Whitney,*** Median, Van Der Waerden, and Savage tests.

For the multi-sample case, the NPAR1WAY Procedure gives exact p-values for the ***Kruskal-Wallis,*** Brown-Mood, k-sample Van Der Waerden, and k-sample Savage tests.

Npar1way is useful when the response variable cannot logically be assumed to be normally distributed.

When data are not normally distributed and the measurements at best contain rank-order information, computing the standard descriptive statistics (e.g., mean, standard deviation) is sometimes not the most informative way to summarize the data.

Parametric tests are often preferred because:

- They are robust
- They have greater power efficiency (greater power relative to the sample size)
- They provide unique information (e.g., the interaction in a factorial design)

Nonparametric methods are most appropriate when the sample sizes are small

What happens when you use a nonparametric test with data from a normal distribution is Greater incidence of Type II error.

- The nonparametric version of analysis of variance is based on ranks.
- The Mann-Whitney test and the Wilcoxon rank sum test are equivalent nonparametric techniques to compare two groups, while the Kruskal-Wallis test is ordinarily used to compare three or more groups.
- All of these are available in PROC NPAR1WAY (nonparametric 1-way analysis of variance) in SAS.

PROC NPAR1WAY performs tests for location and scale differences based on the following scores of a response variable: Wilcoxon, median, Siegel-Tukey and Many more. Additionally, PROC NPAR1WAY provides tests using the raw data as scores. When the data are classified into two samples, tests are based on simple linear rank statistics. When the data are classified into more than two samples, tests are based on one-way ANOVA statistics. Both asymptotic and exact p-values are available for these tests.

PROC NPAR1WAY also calculates the following empirical distribution function (EDF) statistics: the Kolmogorov- Smirnov statistic, when the data are classified into only two samples, the Kuiper statistic. These statistics test whether the distribution of a variable is the same across different groups. When there are two factors with no interaction, as in a randomized complete block design, Friedman's chi-square test is a non-parametric test that can be used to examine treatment differences. Friedman's test is available in SAS under PROC FREQ.

Wilcoxon signed-rank Test

- The Wilcoxon signed-rank test is a non-parametric analog of the one-sample t-test
- The signed-rank test can be used to make inferences about a population mean or median without requiring the assumption of normally distributed data.
- As its name implies, the Wilcoxon signed-rank test is based on the ranks of the data.

- One of the most common applications of the signed-rank test in clinical trials is to compare responses between correlated or paired data, such as testing for significant pre- to post-study changes of a non-normally distributed evaluation measurement.

```
Data Trial;
Input Patid Pre Post @@;
Diff = Pre - post;
Datalines;
1 15 8 2 10 3 3 6 7 4 5 13
5 10 2 6 15 12 7 7 14 8 5 8
9 8 13 10 12 3 11 4 9 12 13 3
13 8 10 14 10 2 15 11 4 16 13 7
17 6 1 18 6 11 19 9 3 20 5 5
21 10 2 22 9 8 23 11 5 24 8 8
;
Run;
Proc Univariate Data = Trial Normal ;
Var Diff;
Run;
```

We perform the above test with Normal Option in the Assumption that the data follows Normal distribution. By considering the Shapiro-Wilk test with p-value of 0.0322, we reject null hypothesis stating that the data is not from Normal distribution.

Now the test of choice is Wilcoxon Signed rank test from Proc Univariate output.

Wilcoxon Rank sum Test

Wilcoxon rank-sum test is a non-parametric analog of the two-sample t-test between two independent populations without the assumption of normally distributed data.

```
Data Trial;
Input Trt $ Response Count @@;
Datalines;
Active 5 5 Active 4 11 Active 3 5 Active 2 1 Active 1 5
Placebo 5 2 Placebo 4 4 Placebo 3 7 Placebo 2 7 Placebo 1 12
;
Run;
```

In the above dataset Trt is a Binomial Variable with two independent populations, Response is an ordinal variable with five ordered (Ranked) values, and if the assumption of normal distribution has not been considered. So we go for Wilcoxon Rank sum Test, by using Proc Npar1way.

```
Proc Npar1way Data=Trial Wilcoxon median;
Class Trt;
Var Response;
Freq Count;
Run;
```

By executing the above Test, we need to consider Pr> |Z| value as P-Value

For skewed distributions with long tails to the right, the median is usually smaller than the mean and considered a better measure of the distributional 'center' or location.

Proc ANOVA (ANOVA Procedure)

ANOVA is used to determine if there is any significant difference between the means of groups of data. There must be at least three groups of data.

For two or more groups, test difference between means, for quantitative normally distributed variables. Just an extension of the t-test (an ANOVA with only two groups is mathematically equivalent to a t-test).

Assumptions of ANOVA:

- Normally distributed outcome
- Equal variances between the groups
- Groups are independent

If we have three groups to compare: we could do three pair-wise ttests, but this would increase our type I error. At an error rate of 5% each test, this means we have an overall chance of up to 1-(.95)3= 14% of making a type-I error (if all 3 comparisons were independent).

In clinical trials, ANOVA method might be appropriate for comparing mean responses among a number of parallel-dose groups or among various strata based on patient's background information, such as Race, Age group, or Disease severity.

```
Data Test;
Input Patid Trt $ Chg_val @@;
Datalines;
101 a 6 102 p 1 103 a 7 104 a 3 105 p 0 106 a 2 107 p 4 108 p 8 109 p 0 110 a 11
111 a 6 112 p 2 113 o 3 114 o 1 115 o 0 116 o 1 117 o 2 118 o 3
;
Run;
```

Now we want to test the significance difference among group means,

The hypotheses are:

- H0: all means are equal,
- HA: not all the means are equal

```
Proc Sort Data=Test;
By Trt;
Run;
```

Here in this dataset we have three values for Trt variable, and the assumption of the continuous variable was normally distributed, since the data is balanced we use ANOVA.

To check whether the data is balanced or not, we need to execute Proc Freq and check the Number of observations for each Trt.

```
Proc Freq Data=Test;
Tables Trt;
Run;

ODS Trace On;
Proc Anova Data=Test;
Class Trt;
Model Chg_val=Trt;
ODS Output OverallANOVA = Anvds;
Run;

ODS trace off;
```

In model statement, Remember to specify Dependent Variable = Independent Variable

- The two-way ANOVA is a method for simultaneously analyzing two factors that affect a response.
- As in the one-way ANOVA, there is a group effect, such as treatment group or dose level. The two-way ANOVA also includes another identifiable source of variation called a blocking factor, whose variation can be separated from the error variation to give more precise group comparisons.
- Because clinical studies often use factors such as study Site, Gender (Sex), diagnostic group, or disease severity as stratification or blocking factor, the two-way ANOVA is one of the most common ANOVA methods used in clinical data analysis.

Kruskal-Wallis test

The Kruskal-Wallis test is a non-parametric analogue of the one-way ANOVA It is used to compare population location parameters (mean, median, etc.) among two or more groups based on independent samples.

The Kruskal- Wallis test is an extension of the Wilcoxon rank-sum test for more than two groups, just as a one-way ANOVA is an extension of the Two-sample Ttest.

The Kruskal-Wallis test is based on the ranks of the data.

This test is often useful in clinical trials for comparing responses among three or more dose groups or treatment groups using samples of non-normally distributed response data.

If Continuous variable is NND (Assumed as Not Normally Distributed) and Categorical variable have greater than or equal to 3 Responses, we use Kruskal Wallis Test.

```
Data Trial;
Input Dose $ Patid Score @@;
Datalines;
1mg 1 5 1mg 6 4 1mg 9 1 1mg 12 2
1mg 15 4 1mg 19 3 1mg 20 6 1mg 23 3
1mg 27 4 1mg 32 1 2mg 35 4 2mg 5 2
2mg 7 2 2mg 10 5 2mg 14 5 2mg 18 4
2mg 22 5 2mg 26 4 2mg 28 3 2mg 31 4
4mg 5 3 4mg 4 3 4mg 8 1 4mg 11 1
4mg 13 2 4mg 16 4 4mg 17 2 4mg 21 1
4mg 24 4 4mg 25 5 4mg 29 4 4mg 30 5
;
Run;
Proc Npar1way Wilcoxon Data=Trial;
Class Dose;
Var Score;
Run;
```

CORR Procedure

When analyzing vast amounts of data, simple statistics can reveal a great deal of information. However, it is often more important to examine relationships within the data, especially in clinical studies. Through correlation measures and hypothesis testing, these relationships can be studied in depth, limited only by the data available in the trial. When examining data in SAS, correlation reveals itself by the relationship between two variables in a dataset. The most common measure of correlation is called the "Pearson Product-Moment Correlation Coefficient".

It is important to note that while more than two variables can be analyzed when looking for correlation, the correlation measure only applies to two variables at a time.

This measure can range from -1 to 1, inclusive. A value of -1 represents a "perfect negative correlation", while a value of 1 represents a "perfect positive correlation". The closer a correlation measure is to these extremes, the "stronger" the correlation between the two variables. A value of zero means that no correlation is observed.

It is important to note that a correlation measure of zero does not necessarily mean that there is no relationship between the two variables, just that there is no linear relationship present in the data that is being analyzed.

It is important to note that a strong (or even perfect) correlation does not imply causation, as other variables may be affecting the relationship between the two variables of interest.

CORRELATION: SYNTAX

In order to measure correlation in SAS, the Proc Corr Procedure can be used. This Procedure will provide correlation measures for multiple variables, in a cross-tabular format.

The syntax for the Procedure is as follows:

Proc Corr Data=DSName;

By byvars;

Freq freqvar;

Var varlist;

Weight weightvar;

Run;

Where:

- DSName is the name of the dataset to be analyzed, either temporary or permanent.
- Byvars is a list of all variables to be used to create 'by' groups for Processing. This option is common among most Procedures.

- Freqvar is the numeric variable which contains the number of times an observation is to be "counted" for the analysis.
- Varlist is a list of all numeric variables to be included in the analysis. At least two numeric variables should be chosen. If no variables are listed, all numeric variables contained in the dataset will be used.
- Weightvar is the numeric variable which contains the weight for each observation. Similar to freqvar.

Data DMVit;

Merge YLP. Dmads (In=indm) YLP.Vitals (In=invit);

By Patid;

If indm and invit;

Run;

Data Vitals;

Set dmvit (keep=patid ageyr vstest vsrn);

Where vstest='hrt';

Run;

Proc Corr Data= Vitals;

Var Vsrn;

With ageyr;

Run;

CORRELATION: OUTPUT

The output produced by Proc Corr contains a great deal of useful information.

- The first information displayed is a list of the variables included in this analysis. This is especially useful when no variables were included in the Var statement, so all numeric variables were included.
- Next is a list of "simple statistics" for each variable. This list contains the number of observations, Mean, Standard deviation, Sum, Minimum and Maximum.
- After this section, each variable in the analysis and their label is listed.

- Finally, the correlation measures are presented. Unless a different correlation measure is requested, this section will be labeled "Pearson Correlation Coefficients".
- Results are provided in a cross-tabular format, with values of one (1) on the diagonal (a variable will always have a perfect positive correlation with itself).
- Along with the correlation coefficients, p-values are listed, as are the number of observations (if different).

In order to test for correlation between HRT and Age, for example, the following code would be used:

Proc Corr data=Vitals;

Var ageyr vsrn;

Run;

The reported correlation measures i.e. 0.884, show a strong positive correlation between age and HRT, but caution must be taken when interpreting these results. Remember, correlation shows linear relationships between two variables, not causation.

Correlation measures may be clouded by relationships that exist with other variables. For example, increasing age may lead to increased convenience food consumption and decreased exercise, which in turn would increase HRT.

Therefore it is not necessarily an increase in age that causes an increase or decrease in HRT, but a change in factors that are related to age. This is known as a "spurious relationship".

By using Proc Corr we can find out the relationship between two variables, by the way of creating and considering R- Value (Rho-Value).

R-Value: Pearson product-moment correlation coefficients. Correlation coefficients are a way of measuring linear relationships between two variables.

Pearson correlation coefficients are useful for continuous variables, while Spearman correlation coefficients are useful for ordinal variables.

The correlation coefficient allows researchers to determine if there is a possible linear relationship between two variables measured on the same subject (or entity). When these two variables are of a continuous nature (they are measurements such as weight, height, length, etc.) the measure of association most often used is Pearson's correlation coefficient.

Regression Analysis

Regression is a statistical Procedure which attempts to predict the values of a given variable, (termed the dependent, outcome, or response variable) based on the values of one or more other variables (called independent variables, predictors, or covariates).

The result of a regression is usually an equation (or model) which summarizes the relationship between the dependent and independent variable(s).

Typically, the model is accompanied by summary statistics describing how well the model fits the data, the amount of variation in the outcome accounted for by the model, and a basis for comparing the existing model to other similar models.

By comparing these statistics across multiple models the user is able to determine a combination and order of independent variables that most satisfactorily predict the values of the outcome.

Linear regression is used to predict the values of a continuous outcome (dependent) variable based on the values of one or more independent predictor variables. Regression analysis is used to analyze the relationship between a response, y, and a quantitative factor, x.

Examples:

- Modeling of blood pressure response (y) on the dose of a new antihypertensive drug (x),
- Cholesterol level (y) on patients age (x),
- Pain relief (y) on time after dosing with an anti-inflammatory treatment (x),
- Degree of wound healing (y) on the baseline surface area of a burn wound (x).

The syntax for the Proc Reg is as follows:

Proc Reg Data=dataset;

By byvars;

*/*Class statement is different when compared to other Procedures */*

Model Depvar=Indepvar(s);

Freq freqvar;

Weight weightvar;

Run;

Quit;

- Dataset is the name of the dataset to be analyzed, either temporary or permanent.
- Byvars is a list of all variables to be used to create "by" groups for Processing. This option is common among most Procedures.
- Depvar is the name of the dependent variable to be used in the analysis (Y).
- Indepvars is a list of all independent variables to be used in the analysis (x1 … xn).
- Freqvar is the numeric variable which contains the number of times an observation is to be "counted" for the analysis. Similar to weightvar.
- Weightvar is the numeric variable which contains the weight for each observation. Similar to freqvar.

Syntax of Proc Reg:

PROC REG DATA=Dataset Options;

MODEL Dependent = Independent(s) / Options;

RUN;

QUIT;

In order to perform regression analysis in SAS, the Proc Reg Procedure can be used. This Procedure will provide regression analysis measures for multiple variables, in a cross-tabular format.

REGRESSION ANALYSIS: EXAMPLE

This example will build on the previous correlation analysis. In order to overcome a possible spurious relationship between BMI and age, variables like food and exercise will be added to the analysis.

Since these variables are now being "controlled" for, the analysis can examine the effect of age independent of the corresponding effects of fast food consumption and lack of exercise.

BMI = ß0 + ß1 + ß2 + ß3

H0: ß1 = 0

Where:

- BMI is the Dependent variable.
- ß0 is referred to as the intercept.
- ß1 ß2 ß3 are the Independent variables.
- H0 is the null hypothesis that the coefficient on the variable age is zero.
- H1 is the alternative hypothesis that the coefficient on the variable age is not zero.In order to test the hypothesis that age has an effect on BMI independent of fast food
- consumption and exercise, the following code would be used:

```
Data Trial;
Input Patid Dur Resp @@;
Label Resp= 'Response in Percent';
Datalines;
1 1 40 2 1 90 3 3 30 4 2 30
5 1 80 6 5 60 7 1 10 8 4 -10
9 2 50 10 6 40 11 1 60 12 4 0
13 2 50 14 2 110 15 3 20 16 3 70
17 5 -30 18 3 20 19 1 40 20 6 0
;
Run;
```

Since the dependent variable is continuous, we go for Proc Reg

```
Proc Reg Data=Trial;
Model Resp=Dur;
Run;
Quit;
```

REGRESSION ANALYSIS: OUTPUT

The output produced by Proc Reg contains a great deal of useful information.

The first information displayed is a count of the observations included in this analysis.

The number of observations "used" in calculating the coefficients is included because missing values for either the dependent or independent variables are excluded from the analysis.

Next is an "Analysis of Variance", including degrees of freedom, sum of squares, and the f value ("Pr > F" shows the probability that all coefficients of the independent variables are equal to zero).Also of interest in this section is the R-square and adjusted R-square values. These values represent the percentage of variation that is being captured by the regression model.

Finally, the parameter estimates (ß0 … ßn) are presented. Along with an estimate of the value, t values are included to test significance ("Pr > |t|" is the probability that a given coefficient is not statistically significant).

```
Proc GLM Data = Trial;
Model Resp = Dur / p clm ss1;
Run;
Quit;
```

Suppose we wish to examine factors that predict patient's hemoglobin levels

```
Data Sample;
Input Patid age race $ BMI Hgb;
Datalines;
21 25 W 18.0 9.3
27 34 W 26.2 11.1
45 21 B 17.9 9.1
12 28 B 22.6 10.5
13 23 W 28.7 11.6
44 32 W 20.4 10.2
;
Run;
```

If we wish to investigate whether BMI can be used to predict hemoglobin levels, we can use simple linear regression. If we wish to investigate whether BMI can be used to predict hemoglobin levels but we also expect age to impact hemoglobin levels, we can use a multiple linear regression to investigate the relationship of both BMI and age with hemoglobin levels.

CAUTION: Sample size is an important consideration when conducting a linear regression. Whenever possible, a sample size calculation should be made prior to data collection. However, we offer as a rule of thumb that the number of observations be at least 10 times the number of predictors.

There are two Procedures in SAS that are typically used to perform linear regression, PROC GLM and PROC REG. We will illustrate the use of PROC GLM to investigate whether BMI can be used to predict hemoglobin levels. The syntax for a simple linear regression is as follows:

```
Proc GLM Data=Sample;
Model Hgb=BMI;
Run;
Quit;
```

For Proc GLM, a quit statement is needed so that Proc GLM will not continue to run in the background.

By default, SAS outputs both the number of observations in the dataset (Number of Observations Read) and the number of observations used in the analysis (Number of Observations Used).

SAS also includes the overall ANOVA table, R-square value, Type I SS analysis, Type III SS analysis, and, for cases where all covariates are continuous, Parameter Estimates.

SAS also includes the overall ANOVA table, R-square value, Type I SS analysis, Type III SS analysis, and, for cases where all covariates are continuous, Parameter Estimates.

Multiple Linear Regressions

The syntax for a multiple linear regression investigating the effects of both BMI and age on hemoglobin levels using PROC GLM is as follows:

```
Proc GLM Data=Sample Plots=none;
Model hgb=bmi age;
Run;
Quit;
```

- As in the simple linear regression case SAS outputs both the number of observations in the dataset (Number of Observations Read) and the number of observations used in the analysis (Number of Observations Used).
- In multiple linear regressions, the R-square value represents the proportion of variability in the outcome explained by the model.
- In this example, approximately 98% of the variability in hemoglobin levels can be explained by the model.
- The Parameter Estimates can be used to determine the regression equation. For this example:
- This means that, holding age constant, we can predict that an increase of one point in BMI will result in a 0.210 increase in hemoglobin level.

LOGISTIC Regression

Logistic regression analysis is a statistical modeling method for analyzing categorical response data while accommodating adjustments for one or more explanatory variables or 'covariates'.

- Linear regression and ANCOVA analyze means of numeric response measures
- Logistic regression analyzes proportions based on categorical responses, most commonly binary responses (e.g., success rates, survival rates, or cure rates).

Examples:

- Comparing survival rates in cancer patients among various treatment groups adjusted for age and duration of disease.
- Comparing proportions of patients whose dermal ulcers show complete healing between an active and placebo group adjusted for baseline ulcer size.
- Comparing the proportion of normalized hypertensive patients between two anti-hypertensive treatment groups adjusted for age, cholesterol level, tobacco use, and exercise habits.

The primary distinction between the REG and LOGISTIC Procedures is that the latter is intended for the modeling of dichotomous categorical outcomes (e.g., dead vs. alive, cancer vs. none…).

```
PROC LOGISTIC DATA=Dataset Options;
CLASS classification variables;
MODEL Dependent = Independent(s) / Options;
RUN;
QUIT;

Data Test;
Input Patid Trt $ Months Relapse $ @@;
Datalines;
101 ACT 3 NO 102 PBO 3 YES 104 ACT 3 YES
106 ACT 6 YES 107 ACT 5 NO 110 ACT 6 YES
111 ACT 6 YES 114 PBO 6 YES 115 ACT 15 NO
117 ACT 15 NO 120 ACT 12 NO 121 ACT 18 NO
122 ACT 6 YES 125 ACT 15 NO 126 PBO 6 YES
128 ACT 15 NO 129 ACT 12 YES 132 ACT 9 NO
133 PBO 6 YES 136 PBO 6 NO 139 ACT 6 NO
142 ACT 6 NO 144 PBO 3 YES 146 ACT 18 NO
149 ACT 9 NO 150 ACT 12 YES 152 ACT 6 NO
154 ACT 9 YES 156 ACT 9 YES 158 PBO 3 NO
;
Run;

Proc Logistic Data=Test  descending;
Class Trt (Ref='PBO');
Model relapse (event='YES')= trt months;
Run;

Proc freq Data = Test;
Tables trt*relapse / chisq nocol nopercent nocum;
Run;
```

It always seems impossible until it is done.

Nelson Mandela

STEP 11

SAS MACROS

SAS Macros can accomplish repetitive tasks quickly and efficiently. Whenever you find yourself writing similar code over and over again, then macros may make your job easier. The macro facility is a tool for text substitution, which reduces the amount of text entered for common tasks. The SAS Macro language can make programming easier and more fun, if used properly.

Advantages of SAS Macro Facility:

- Avoid repetitious SAS code
- Create reusable and flexible SAS code
- Pass information from one part of a SAS job to another
- Conditionally execute data steps and PROCs
- Dynamically create code at execution time

Macros has two basic building blocks: Macros (Macro Programs) and Macro Variables.

Macro always uses two symbols known as macro triggers i.e. & and %. Macro Variables start with an ampersand (&), and names of macros start with a percent sign (%).

Macro Program → Starts with % followed by a Character or _ (Underscore) like %Chd, %_Ch

Macro Variable → Starts with & followed by a Character or _ (Underscore) like &Chd, &_Ch

Macro terminology

- Input stack: Holds a SAS program after it is submitted and before it is processed by the word scanner.

- Word scanner: Scans the text it takes from the input stack and breaks the text into tokens, determines the destination of the token: DATA step compiler, macro Processor, etc.
- Token: Fundamental unit in the SAS language. SAS statements must be broken down into tokens, or tokenized, before the statements can be compiled. Tokens are the actual words in the SAS statements as well as the literal strings, numbers, and symbols.
- Compiler: Checks the syntax of tokens received from the word scanner. After it completes checking the syntax, the compiler translates the tokens into a form for execution.
- Macro Processor: Processes macro language references and statements.
- Macro trigger: The symbols & and %, when followed by a letter or underscore, that signal the word scanner to transfer what follows to the macro Processor.
- Macro symbol table: The area in memory where macro variables and their associated Values are stored.

Macro Variables

Macro variables are tools that allow you to write reusable programs. A macro variable does not belong to a data set and has only a single Value which is always character. The Value of a macro variable could be a variable name, a numeral, or text.

Characteristics of macro variables:

- A macro variable can be referenced anywhere in a SAS program other than in data lines.
- Macro variables names must be a Valid SAS name and start with a letter or underscore.
- They can be used in either open code or inside a macro definition or program.
- Macro variables are not dataset variables and do not relate directly to observations in a dataset, they are tools that allow you to write reusable code.
- Macro variables can be stored in either the global symbol table or in a local symbol table.

- Macro variable Values are text Values.
- Macro variables are not data set variables, and their purpose is different from data set variables.

There are two types of macro variables, 1) Automatic 2) User-defined:

- Automatic macro variables are defined by the SAS system at the start of each session. Most automatic variables contain information about your session, such as date, time when session opened, version, etc.
- User-defined macro variables are defined by the programmer and are specific to the programmers needs.

There are two types of User-defined macro variables.

- Local macro variables
- Global macro variables

Local: Variables defined inside the macro definition are considered to be local variables.

Global: Variables defined outside the macro definition, or inside the macro specified as global, are considered to be global variables.

Different ways of creating macro variables:

- %Let statement
- Iterative %DO statement
- %GLOBAL statement
- %INPUT statement
- INTO clause in Proc/SQL
- %LOCAL statement
- %MACRO statement
- SYMPUT routine and SYMPUTN routine (Call Routine)

%LET Statement:

%Let is a GLOBAL statement. It can occur anywhere within a SAS job, i.e. it is not restricted to DATA steps (or PROCs).

The %Let statement is written as follows and is terminated with a semicolon.

%Let macro-variable-name = macro-variable-Value;

Creating a Macro Variable in open code

%Let Prog = T_1_1;

- By executing the above statement, we created macro variable Prog which is stored in global symbol table.
- No quotation marks are required to enclose the macro variable Value. If quotation marks are used, they become part of the Value.
- Once the macro variable is defined, you must precede the name of the macro variable with an ampersand (&) each time it is used.

The %Put statement writes text and the current Values of macro variables to the SAS system LOG.

Syntax:

%Put &Macro-Variable-list;

Options available for the %Put statement as listed below:

- _All_: Lists all macro variables in all referencing environments.
- _Automatic_: Lists all the macro variables that are automatically defined at your site.
- _Global_: Lists all the user-created global macro variables that are available.

%Put _User_;

By executing above statement we can obtain the list of user defined macro variables in the log window

If a macro variable appears within a quoted string (e.g. Title, Footnote, Note), double quotes must be used to ensure that the macro variable 'resolves' to its assigned Value.

Resolving a macro variable

A macro variable defined inside or outside the macro is referred by prefixing an ampersand (&) before its name.

Using macro variables wrongly:

Title '&Prog' created on '&Sysdate';

Proc Print Data=YLP.Demog;

Run;

Using macro variables in the right way

Title "&Prog" created on "&Sysdate9";

Proc Print Data=YLP.Demog;

Run;

Placing text before macro variable reference

%Let FValue=3;

%Let SValue=12;

Data Lab&FValue&SValue;→It resolves to Lab312;

Placing text after macro variable reference

%Let Lib=YLP;

%Let Dsn=Demog;

Data &Lib.&Dsn;

It resolves to YLPDemog but we are expecting YLP.Demog, this is because, the macro Processor sends the macro variable references back to the input stack as they were received. The word scanner cannot tokenize the data statement so we use proper delimiters to perform this like the following:

Data &Lib..&Dsn;

%Let Lib=YLP;

%Let Dsn=AE;

Wrong usage of Lib as well as Dsn name

Data &Lib. &Dsn;

Set YLP.Events;

Run;

Correct usage

Data &Lib..&Dsn;

Set YLP.Events;

Run;

Referencing macro variables indirectly

When two or more ampersands (&) appear next to each other, successive passes or scans are required to make the final resolution. You can think of the double ampersand (&&) as a special reference that resolves to a single ampersand.

The rules that the macro Processor uses to resolve macro variable references that contain multiple ampersands follow.

- Macro variable references are resolved from left to right.
- Two ampersands (&&) resolve to one ampersand (&).
- Multiple leading ampersands cause the macro Processor to rescan the reference until no more ampersands can be resolved.

  %Let SAS=CLINITRIAL;

  %Let YLP38=SAS;

  %Let Name=YLP;

  %Let Age=38;

Wrong calling of two macro variables in a sequence

%Put &&Name&Age;

*%Let Value=&&name&age; *Incorrect Indirect Reference;*

WARNING: Apparent symbolic reference NAME38 not resolved.

The above resolution would not happen as per expectation because Macro Processor is scanning the text for two passes

Correct usage

*%Let Value=&&&name&age;*Correct Indirect Reference;*

%Put &&&Name&Age; → *SAS*

Note: to obtain CLINITRIAL, we need to give 7 ampersands before Name&Age. *%Put &&&&&&&Name&Age;* → *CLINITRIAL*
Written test Question: *%Let X= 15;* *%Macro Test;* *%Let X=10;* *%put X inside macro Test= &X;* *%Mend Test;* *%Test;* *What would you see in the log window, if you execute the below statements:* ✦ *%Put X outside Macro Test=&X;* ✦ *%Put X inside Macro Test=&X;*

Creating Macro variables from Data step

CALL SYMPUT ROUTINE:

Call Symput Assigns DATA step information to a macro variable (Information obtained from one datastep would be assigned to a macro variable and used where ever it is required). The variables created by call Symput are global.

Syntax:

CALL SYMPUT (Argument-1, Argument-2);

- ***Argument-1:*** Specifies a character expression that identifies the macro variable that is assigned a Value. If the macro variable does not exist, the routine creates it.
- ***Argument-2:*** Specifies a character constant, variable, or expression that contains the Value that is assigned.

```
Data Demog;
Set YLP. Demog  End=EOF;  *End Of File;
If Sex=1 Then Cntone+1;
Else If Sex=2 Then Cnttwo+1;
Cnttot+1;
If EOF Then
        Do;
            Call Symput ('N1', Put (cntone, 4.));
            Call Symput ('N2', Put (cnttwo, 4.));
            Call Symput ('Nt', Put (Cnttot, 4.));
        End;
Run;
```

CALL SYMPUTX ROUTINE

The CALL SYMPUTX routine is a quick and simple way to store or assign Values into macro variables. Once stored, these Values can be accessed globally throughout a program and can be displayed in generated reports.

Syntax:

Call Symputx (Macro-variable, Value);

The macro-variable argument can be:

a) A character string in quotation marks b) A character variable name

Values of the macro-variable argument must follow existing naming rules for macro variables.

The Value argument can be:

a) A character or numeric Value b) A character or numeric variable name

Note: When using the CALL SYMPUTX routine, all leading and trailing spaces are truncated from both the macro-variable and the Value.

The CALL SYMPUTX routine can be used repeatedly, at any point in the DATA step.

EXAMPLE 1: CALL SYMPUTX

In this example we will create a macro variable named &Year which will store the numeric Value of 2014 and the macro variable named &Trt1 which will store the character Value of "Placebo".

```
Data _null_;
        Call Symputx ('Year', 2014);
        Call Symputx ('Trt1', 'Placebo');
Run;
```

A %PUT statement will show the Value of &Year and &Trt1.

%Put &Year &Trt1; → The log result displays: 2014 Placebo

> ***Written test Question***
>
> ```
> %Macro Test;
> %LOCAL Value2;
> Data _null_;
> Call Symput ('Value1','20');
> Run;
> %Let Value2 = 100;
> %Mend Test;
> %Test;
> %Put A = &Value1  B = &Value2;
> ```
>
> *What would be the output of %PUT statement?*

Symget and Symgetn Functions

The SYMGET and SYMGETN functions easily retrieve the Values of previously stored macro variables and assign these Values in new User defined variables. The choice of SYMGET or SYMGETN is dictated by the data type of the original macro variable Value.

SYMGET is used to store character Values, while numeric Values require SYMGETN.

→ With SYMGET, the programmer-defined variable will be a character string;

Retrieving a character Value from the given macro-variable:

- ✦ Variable = Symget ('Macro-variable');
- → With SYMGETN, the programmer-defined variable will be numeric;

Retrieving a numeric Value from the given macro-variable:

- ✦ Variable = Symgetn ('macro-variable');

As with the CALL SYMPUT routine, the macro-variable for both SYMGET and SYMGETN can either be:

- ✦ The name of a macro variable with no ampersand (within the single quotation marks)
- ✦ The name of a variable with Values that have been assigned as macro variables.

Let's recall our example of the CALL SYMPUT routine where we assigned the macro variable &Year with the numeric Value 2014. We now want to create a new variable called Cur_Year that will be assigned the Value of &Year.

Executing the following code will produce the dataset, DSET2, as displayed below:

```
Data Dsn;
Cur_Year = Symgetn ('Year');
Run;
```

A PRACTICAL EXAMPLE COMBINING CALL SYMPUT AND SYMGETN

Consider the following dataset:

- ✦ TREAT is a character variable with Values of either "A" or "B".
- ✦ GENDER is also character variable with Values of either "Male" or "Female".
- ✦ USUBJID is a numeric unique subject identifier variable.

Suppose we want to calculate the number and percentage of subjects by gender for each treatment group. First we count the number of subjects in each treatment group; this is accomplished through use of the PROC FREQ. This result will serve as our denominator:

```
Data Demog;
Input Subjid Treat $ Gender $@@ ;
Datalines;
101 Active Male 102 Placebo Female 103 Active Female 104 Placebo Male
105 Placebo Male 106 Active Female 107 Active Male 108 Active Female
109 Active Male 110 Active Female 111 Placebo Male 112 Active Female
113 Placebo Male 114 Active Female 115 Active Male 116 Active Female
;
Run;

Proc Freq Data=Demog Noprint;
Tables Treat / Out=Trtfreq;
Run;
```

The dataset TRTFREQ created. There are 5 subjects assigned to Treatment Placebo and 11subjects assigned to Treatment Active.

Using the CALL SYMPUT routine, we assign macro variables for the Value of TREAT.

```
Data _Null_;
Set Trtfreq;
Call Symputx (Treat, Count);
Run;

%Put _User_;
```

We now have the macro variable &Active, which contains the Value of 11, and the macro variable &Placebo, which contains the Value 5. Both &Active and &Placebo are numeric because COUNT is numeric. We now have our denominators for both treatment groups stored in macro variables.

To obtain the number of "Male" and "Female" subjects by Treatment Group, we will again use PROC FREQ.

```
Proc Freq Data=Demog Noprint;
Tables Treat*Gender / Out=genfreq (Drop=Percent);
Run;
```

To calculate the percentages of male and female subjects in each treatment group, we divide COUNT by the number of subjects in each treatment group.

```
Data Final;
Set genfreq;
Percent=Count/Symgetn (Treat)*100;
Run;
```

The dataset FINAL is created with the new variable PERCENT.

Building a better Macro

Even though the macro facility has great power, it is often misused by the programmers. So, while creating a macro program we need to consider the following points:

I. Check whether the macro is necessary in that specific situation or not

- Repetitive tasks
- Conditional execution of program fragments
- Tasks that have varying execution paths and thus need to be parameterized

II. Conceptually Separate Utilities and Applications

Examples of macro utilities:

- Count the number of observations in a data set
- Convert one or more macro variables to upper case
- Create a count and list of distinct Values of a data sets variable
- Quote each token in a macro variable
- Check for the presence of one or more variables in a data set

Examples of macro applications:

- Print the first "n" observations for every data set in a library.
- Create a set of PDF files that display attributes for data sets and variables in a library.
- Check the contents of one or more data sets for compliance with internal or external (legal, industry) standards.

III. Clearly Document the Macro:

This is usually placed in a comment at the beginning of the Macro, This list identifies some common features:

- Macro name
- Description
- Inputs
- Outputs
- Processing
- Execution
- Error conditions
- History of the macro

IV. Use Keyword Parameters Consistently:

As per our SOP we should always use keyword parameters rather than positional parameters. If we use keyword parameters, user doesn't have to worry about parameter order, and the program becomes somewhat self-documenting by having parameters and their Values present in the call to that specific macro.

V. Use Consistent Program Structure:

In general terms, a macro should consist of four sections:

1. Header Documentation
2. Initialization:
    - verifying correct execution environment,
    - checking parameters and resources,
    - capturing Values of options that will be reset,
    - defining local and global macro variables,
    - converting parameters to upper case
3. Core Processing
4. Termination: Deleting temporary macro variables, files, and data sets, resetting options back to their original Values, writing messages to the SAS Log

VI. Control Macro Variable Scope:

VII. Implement Diagnostic and Debugging Code

IX: Validation:

- Confirm there is adequate header documentation
- Verify macro output is limited to what was described in the header comment
- Examine naming and default Values of keyword parameters, ensuring they match what is described in header comment
- Thoroughly test parameter error-checking
- Examine the program for appropriate exception/error handling
- Confirm that the termination section removes temporary variables, datasets, etc. and sets any re-set options to their original state.

Macro Parameters

Macro parameters allow you to define macro variables. Macro parameters are used to pass Values or text strings into a macro.

Types of Macro Parameters

- Positional parameters
- Keyword (named) parameters

Positional parameters

- Positional parameters derive their name from the fact that they are defined using a specific position on the %Macro statement.
- When a macro is executed, the Value is passed using that same position in the macro call.

Keyword parameters

- Parameters may be designated as keywords in the %Macro statement.
- Keyword parameters may be used in any order and may be assigned default Values.
- Keyword parameters are designated by following the parameter name with an equal sign (=).

Deleting User - Defined Macro Variables

The ***%Symdel statement*** deletes user defined macro variables.

Syntax: %Symdel Macro-Variable-list;

Steps in Creating Macro

- Write the code in BASE SAS, Execute it and check the output, as per expectations or not
- Check for the objects (Datasets, Variables, and Options) which we need to change.
- Plan a MACRO program with these objects as Keyword parameters.
- Create a Macro program.
- Execute the MACRO Program and check for the results.
- Whenever we need to create any report look like this, Modify or Alter some objects in a Macro and execute without altering the Macro Program.

1. Write the code in BASE SAS, execute it and check the output, as per expectations or not

```
Proc sort Data=YLP.Demog Out=Demsrt Nodup;
By Descending Race;
Run;
```

2. Check for the objects which are going to be changed.

- Input Dataset Name
- Output Dataset Name
- Options
- Byopt
- Byvar

3. Plan a MACRO program with the objects as keyword parameters.

```
%macro Sortmac (inds=,otds=,opt=,byopt=,byvar=);
```

4. Create a Macro program.

%Macro Sortmac (inds=,otds=,opt=,byopt=,byvar=);

Proc Sort data=&inds out=&otds &opt;

by &byopt &byvar;

Run;

%Mend sortmac;

5. Execute the MACRO Program and check for the results.

Calling a Macro:

%Sortmac (inds=YLP.Demog, otds=dem, byvar=Race)

%Sortmac(inds=YLP.Dmads, otds=agesrt, byopt=descending, byvar=ageyr)

%Sortmac(inds=YLP.ae, otds=aes, byopt=descending, byvar=aerel)

6. Modify or Alter some variables in a Macro calling and execute the Macro without altering the Macro Program.

Macro Functions

Macro functions are used to create, modify, and work with text strings. Initially this may seem like a minor difference, but because macro functions deal with text, they can be used to build SAS code.

The arguments of a macro function can be text strings, macro variables, macro functions, and macro program calls. The result of a macro function is always text.

We can classify the macro functions into different categories:

- Character → %Index, %Scan, %Substr, %Upcase, %Length
- Evaluation → %Eval, %Sysevalf
- Quoting → %Str, %Nrstr, %Bquote, %Nrbquote, %Quote, %Superq, %Unquote
- Macro variable attribute %Symexist, %Symglobl, %Symlocal
- Other Functions → %Sysfunc, %Qsysfunc

MACRO CHARACTER FUNCTIONS

Macro character functions either change or provide information about the text string that is included as one of the arguments. Many of these functions are analogous to similar functions in the DATA step.

The difference between macro functions and their DATA step equivalents is DATA step functions work on character strings, numeric values, and DATA step variable values. Macro functions are applied to text strings that NEVER contain the values of DATA step variables.

Several of these functions have two forms, with and without a Q at the start of the function name. Functions with names that start with Q (quoting) remove the meaning from special characters including the ampersand (&), percent sign (%), and mnemonic operators in returned values.

%INDEX Function:

Returns the position in source of the first character of string.

Syntax:

%INDEX (source, string);

```
%LET X=Clinical SAS Programmer;
%LET Y=%INDEX (&X, SAS);
%PUT SAS found at position &Y;
```

%SUBSTR Function:

Extracts substring of length characters from argument starting at position.

Syntax:

%SUBSTR (argument, position<, length>);

```
%LET Str= SAS Clinical Programmer;
%LET Part=%SUBSTR (&Str, 1, 3);
%PUT  &Part;
```

%SCAN Function:

Returns the nth word in argument where the words in argument are separated by delimiters.

Syntax

%SCAN (argument, n <, delimiters>)

```
%LET Mob_Num=897 878 4848;
%LET LFD=%SCAN(&Mob_Num,3);
```

%PUT Last Four Digits of the Mobile Number is &LFD;

%UPCASE Function

Converts character string or text expression to uppercase

Syntax:

%UPCASE(string)

```
%LET Str= SAS Clinical Programmer;
%LET Caps=%UPCASE (&Str);
%PUT  &Caps;
```

%LENGTH Function:

This function Returns length of string, of resolute text expression.

Syntax

%LENGTH (string);

```
%MACRO Check (dsn);
%if %LENGTH(&dsn) gt 8 %then
%put Name is too long - &dsn;
%else %do;
Proc Contents Data=&dsn;
Run;
%end;
%MEND Check;
%Check (Disposition)
```

MACRO EVALUATION FUNCTIONS:

- Since in the macro language there are no numbers or numeric variables numeric operations such as arithmetic and logical comparisons become problematic. Evaluation functions are used to bridge the gap between text and numeric operations.

- Macro evaluation functions evaluate arithmetic expressions and logical expressions. The arguments of these macro evaluation functions are temporarily converted to numbers so that a calculation can be completed. The macro evaluation function converts the result that it returns to text.

%EVAL Function

The %EVAL function always performs integer arithmetic. Regardless of the requested operation the result will always be an integer. This function treats numbers with decimal points as text. The %EVAL function generates an error when there is text in the arguments.

Syntax:

%EVAL (arithmetic expression| logical expression)

%Let A=22;

%Let B=&X+11;

%Let C=%EVAL (&X+11);

%Put &A &B &C;

Non-integer arithmetic is not allowed. Check the following statement

%Let D=%EVAL(&A+11.2);

It would result an error being printed in the LOG.

%SYSEVALF function

This function can be used to perform non-integer arithmetic.

Syntax:

%SYSEVALF (arithmetic expression| logical expression <, Conversion-Type>);

- The Expression is any arithmetic or logical expression which is to be evaluated and it may contain macro references.
- The Conversion Type, is an optional conversion to apply to the value returned by %SYSEVALF.
- Conversion Type, can be: Boolean, Ceil, Floor, Integer.

%Let SE=%Sysevalf (33.2 + 44.1);

%Let SI=%Sysevalf (33.2 + 44.1, Integer);

%Put &SE &SI;

MACRO QUOTING FUNCTIONS:

Macro quoting functions mask special characters and mnemonic operators in your macro language statements so that the macro Processor does not interpret them. The macro Processor instead treats these items simply as text.

Quoting functions allow the user to pass macro arguments while selectively removing the special meaning from characters such as &, %, ;, ‘, .

%STR Function:

Often it is used along with the %LET statement to mask semicolons that would otherwise terminate the %LET.

%Let Prg= Data Test; x=5;Run;

%Let Msk_Prg= %STR (Data Test; x=5;Run;);

%put &Msk_Prg;

%BQUOTE Function:

The %BQUOTE function is probably the best choice in quoting functions. It eliminates many of the limitations of the %STR function and it will also remove the meaning from unmatched symbols that are normally found in pairs such as quotes and parentheses.

The following %LET will cause all sorts of problems because the apostrophe will be interpreted as an unmatched quote.

%let Test = Y L Prasad’s SAS Book;

The %STR function will not help because %STR does not mask quote marks, however %BQUOTE does.

%let Q_Test = %BQUOTE (Y L Prasad’s SAS Book);

%put & Q_Test;

%NRSTR Function:

%Let Org=Johnson&Johnson ltd;

By executing the above statement we can observe the WARNING: Apparent symbolic reference Johnson not resolved, this is because SAS Interprets &Johnson as a macro variable rather than simply text.

You must use a macro quoting function (%NRSTR) to tell the macro Processor to ignore the special meaning of the ampersands and percent signs and instead treat them as text

```
%Let Msk_Org=%NRSTR (Johnson&Johnson ltd);
%put &Msk_Org;
Title "Report on &Msk_Org";
Proc Print Data=YLP.Demog;
Run;
```

%SYSFUNC function:

%Sysfunc makes many common macro tasks much simpler and more efficient.This function brings some functionality to macros that was previously available only in the DATA step

Syntax: %SYSFUNC (function (argument(s)) < format >);

The %SYSFUNC function allows the user to execute functions that were previously unavailable in the macro facility , is especially useful in finding information about data sets .while using some functions in macros they might not be resolved, as SAS thinks we are assigning a Value to a macro variable.

Wrong usage of INT function

```
%Let a=33.6;
%Let b=INT(&a);
%put b=&b;
```

Correct usage of INT function

```
%Let a=33.6;
%Let b=%Sysfunc (Int(&a));
%put b=&b;
```

Macro Debugging

Debugging is a Process by which coding errors in a computer program are identified and corrected through a sequence of activities, each of which must be adapted according to the outcomes of the preceding steps.

We can minimize errors in our SAS programs that contain macro features by developing your programs in steps. When your programs do end up containing errors, you can use the tools like system options, macro language statements, macro functions, and automatic macro variables to find the sources of the errors

Using SAS System Options to Debug Macro Programming:

Several system options can provide detail about the Processing of your SAS programs that contain macro language and, thus, help you find the sources of errors in your programs.

1. ***MERROR | Nomerror***

- ✦ When this option is ON SAS will issue a warning message when you are invoking a Macro Program that SAS cannot find.

2. ***SERROR | Noserror***

- ✦ When this option is ON SAS will issue a warning message when you use a Macro Variable that SAS cannot find.

3. ***Mlogic | NOMLOGIC***

- ✦ Traces the flow of execution of a macro program in the SAS log. MLOGIC shows the resolved values of macro parameters, the scope of macro variables (global or local), the true/false result of %IF statements, and the start and end of a macro program.
- ✦ Mlogic traces the macro logic and follows the pattern of execution. The resolved result of a %IF statement is displayed in the LOG as true or false.

4. ***Mprint | NOMPRINT***

- ✦ Displays the SAS code generated by the execution of a macro program in the SAS log. Optionally, you can direct the output from MPRINT to an external file by specifying the MFILE system option.
- ✦ SAS code that is generated by a macro is generally not displayed in the LOG. The Mprint option displays the text or SAS statements that are generated by macro execution, one statement per line.

5. ***Symbolgen | NOSYMBOLGEN***

- ✦ When SYMBOLGEN option is ON SAS prints the Values of MACRO VARIABLES in the LOG Window.

If we want to invoke new messages we can use MPRINT MLOGIC and SYMBOLGEN but we are not supposed to use NOMERROR and NOSERROR as per our SOP.

To present the execution of the macro program and its resolution in the log window

Options Mlogic;

To present the macro variables resolution and their Values in log window

Options Symbolgen;

Options Mprint Symbolgen Mlogic;

%infmac(lib=work,dsn=jag,path='E:\all files\all txt files\data txt files\dem.txt',var= id trt$ age)

To suppress the Mprint option

Options Nomprint;

MFILE Option

MFILE option can be used to write out the resolved macro code to a file. To take advantage of this option, use a FILENAME statement with a Fileref of MPRINT, and turn on both the MPRINT and MFILE options.

FILENAME MPRINT 'D: \Mymacs\Macprog.sas;

Storing Macros

Macros are stored in the work library by default.

There are three types of macro libraries;

- %INCLUDE
- Compiled Stored Macros
- AUTOCALL Macros.

Macro libraries allow the macro developer to store, maintain, and manage large numbers of macros. The two types of macro libraries (AUTOCALL and Compiled Stored Macros), are often used to avoid the use of the %INCLUDE statement to bring in macro definitions.

%INCLUDE does not actually set up a macro library. The %INCLUDE statement points to a file and when the statement is executed, the indicated file is inserted into the calling program at the location of the call. When using the %INCLUDE to build a macro library, the included file will usually contain one or more macro definitions.

COMPILED STORED MACROS

Macros are always compiled before they are executed and it is possible to store the compiled code for future use. Compiled macros are stored in a catalog named SASMACR, and by default this catalog is stored in the WORK library. Each compiled macro is stored with the entry type of MACRO and with an entry name corresponding to the name of the macro. When a macro is called, SAS automatically searches this catalog for the compiled version of the macro that was called. Permanently compiled stored macros are also written to a SASMACR catalog, but this catalog is stored in a different (permanent) library.

The ability to store and make use of compiled stored macros is by default turned off. The user turns on the ability to make use of compiled stored macros with the system option MSTORED (NOMSTORED turns it off). The library that is to be used to store the permanent SASMACR catalog is specified by using the SASMSTORE= option.

The following OPTIONS statement turns on the use of compiled stored macros and designates the YLPMAC libref as the catalog location.

Options Mstored Sasmstore = Ylpmac;

The Mstored system option enables storage of compiled macros in a permanent SAS library

Syntax

Options Mstored Sasmstore=libref;

Process of storing a macro

1. Create a library in which we can store the macro catalog

   Libname Maclib 'E:\mymacros';

2. ***Mention Mstored option*** to specify that we are using stored compiled macro facility use ***Sasmstore= option*** to specify the library name in which we are going to store our macro catalog.

   Options Mstored Sasmstore=Maclib;

3. Use STORE option to mention that we are going to store the macro program

   %MACRO Infmac(dsn=,path=,opt=,var=)/ ***STORE;***

   ----Macro Program----

   %MEND infmac;

4. Calling a stored macro

   Libname maclib 'E:\mymacros';

   Options mstored sasmstore=maclib;

   %Infmac(dsn=dem2, path='E:\data txt files\comdlm.txt', opt=dlm=',', var=id trt$ ae$)

You have to dream before your
dreams can come true

A P J Abdul Kalam

STEP 12

PROC SQL

- PROC SQL is SAS implementation of structured query language. PROC SQL can Sort, Summarize, Subset, Join (merge), and Concatenate datasets, Create new variables, and Print the results or Create a new table or View - all in one step.
- The SQL Procedure is a powerful addition to a SAS programmers, it should not be viewed as a replacement to standard SAS code but as another potential solution.
- PROC SQL can be used to Retrieve, Update, and Report on information from SAS data sets. PROC SQL can often retrieve information with fewer and shorter statements than traditional SAS code. Additionally, SQL often uses fewer resources than conventional DATA and PROC steps.

Applications of Proc SQL in Clinical Programming:

- To create Reports
- To create Macro Variables
- To obtain Summary Statistics
- To Retrieve data from one or more than one table

SQL Terminology

Data Processing	SAS	SQL equivalent
File	SAS dataset	Table
Record	Observation	Row
Field	Variable	Column

Basic Syntax of Proc SQL:

PROC SQL;

SELECT Column, Column . . .

FROM Tablename| Viewname. . .

WHERE Condition...

QUIT;

Syntax Rules in PROC SQL:

- Statements (clauses) in the SQL Procedure are not separated by semicolons, the entire query is terminated with a semicolon.
- Items in an SQL statement are separated by a comma.
- There is a required order of statements in a query.
- One SQL Procedure can contain many queries and a query can reference the results from previous queries.
- The SQL Procedure can be terminated with a QUIT statement, RUN statements have no effect.

SELECT Clause:

- To retrieve and display data a SELECT statement is used.
- The data will be displayed in the order you list the columns in the SELECT statement.
- A column can be a variable, calculated value or formatted value.
- An asterisk (*) can be used to select all columns.

THE SELECT STATEMENT SYNTAX:

- The purpose of the SELECT statement is to describe how the report will look. It consists of the SELECT clause and several sub-clauses. The sub-clauses name the input dataset, select rows meeting certain conditions (Subsetting), group (or aggregate) the data, and order (or sort) the data:

```
PROC SQL options;
        SELECT column(s)
        FROM table-name | view-name
        WHERE expression
        GROUP BY column(s)
        HAVING expression
        ORDER BY column(s);
QUIT;
```

FROM Clause:

✦ The FROM Clause specifies the Input table or tables.

Selecting single column from a table:

```
Proc SQL;
SELECT Patid FROM YLP.Demog;
Quit;
```

> **Note:** Select Clause and From Clause are required Clauses in Select Statement.

Selecting multiple columns from a table:

```
Proc SQL;
        Select Patid, Race from YLP.Demog;
Quit;
```

Selecting all columns:

```
Proc SQL;
        Select * from YLP.Demog;
Quit;
```

Selecting Rows with a WHERE Clause:

✦ The WHERE clause specifies rows to be selected for the query.

We would like to select the race, Ageyr from the Dmads table where the age is less than 50 years.

```
Proc SQL;
Select Race, Ageyr From YLP.Dmads
Where Race = 1 and Ageyr LT 50;
Quit;
```

> **Note:** For the List of where clause operators check Where statement in Proc Print

Ordering the Output with ORDER Clause:

The ORDER clause is used to sequence data for output.

```
Proc SQL;
        Select Patid, Sex, Ageyr
        From YLP. Dmads
        Where Ageyr GT 50 and Sex=1
        ORDER BY Ageyr;
Quit;
```

To arrange data in descending order

```
Proc SQL;
        Select Patid, Sex, Ageyr
        From YLP.Dmads
        Where Ageyr gt 50 and Sex=1
        Order by Ageyr DESC;
Quit;
```

Case Logic:

Case logic is used when you would like to assign specific values based on some criteria. It is used in place of conditional IF statements in SQL. The case statement can compare to a single value or an expression and returns a single value for each condition met.

Syntax:

CASE [operand]

WHEN [condition] THEN [result]

[WHEN condition THEN result] ...

[ELSE result]

END [AS column]

If a CASE operand is specified, the WHEN condition must be an equality. If a CASE operand is not specified, the WHEN condition must be a valid Boolean expression. The result can be a single value or another CASE statement (nested CASE).

Summary Functions:

Summary functions summarize column values for all rows in a table producing an aggregate value. Rows will be summarized to the lowest logical summary. If all columns on the SELECT statement are summary functions then the summary will be based upon all rows in the table.

We would like to show the Average Age, Minimum Age, and Maximum Age, for the Subjects in Dmads table.

```
PROC SQL;
        SELECT AVG (Ageyr) AS Meanage,
        MIN (Ageyr) AS Minage,
        MAX (Ageyr) AS Maxage
        FROM YLP.Dmads;
QUIT;
```

When summary functions and detail values are used in the SELECT statement without a GROUP BY, the summary will be for the entire table although each detail row will be displayed. In this case we are seeing a row for each Subject.

- ✦ To summarize and display data in groups, use a ***GROUP BY clause*** with column functions.
- ✦ To arrange results in a particular order (ascending or descending) use an ***ORDER BY Clause***.

```
Proc SQL;
Select Avg(Ageyr) AS Meanage,
Min (Ageyr) AS Minage,
Max (Ageyr) AS Maxage FROM YLP.Dmads
Group By Race
Order By Meanage Desc;
Quit;
```

We can also choose to display rows by selecting on summary values. This requires the use of the HAVING expression. The HAVING expression follows the GROUP BY clause.

```
Proc SQL;
Select Race, Ageyr
From YLP.Dmads
Group By Race
Having Race in (1,3);
Quit;
```

Creating Tables:

We can create a new table (SAS data set) with the results. The ***CREATE statement*** is used to create SQL tables as a permanent or temporary SAS data sets with the SELECT clause providing the variable list.

```
Proc SQL;
        CREATE Table Test AS
        Select Patid, Sex, Ageyr
        From YLP.Dmads
        Where Ageyr gt 50 and Sex=1
        Order by Ageyr Desc;
Quit;
```

The NOPRINT statement disables output to the SAS output device. (When using a CREATE statement NOPRINT is the default).

CREATING NEW VARIABLES

Variables can be dynamically created in PROC SQL. Dynamically created variables can be given a variable name, label, or neither. If a dynamically created variable is not given a name or a label, it will appear on the report as a column with no column heading.

USING LABELS AND FORMATS

SAS-defined or user-defined formats can be used to improve the appearance of the body of a report. LABELs give the ability to define longer column headings:

```
Data Temp;
Input fn @@;
Datalines;
89 99 98 102 106 67 75 110
78 98 65 67 107 76 54 68
;
Run;
Proc SQL;
        Create Table New_temp as
        Select fn, (fn - 32)* 5/9 as centi Format= 5.2 Label=
        'centgr'
        From Temp;
Quit;
Proc Print Data=New_temp Label;
Run;
```

To determine the structure of a table we use Describe Statement

```
Proc SQL;
        DESCRIBE Table YLP.Events;
Quit;
```

To Replacing missing values we use COALESCE Clause

```
Proc SQL;
        Select Patid, COALESCE (Sex, 999) AS Gender
        From YLP.Demog;
Quit;
```

Using Wildcard Characters for Searching:

When searching for specific rows of data is necessary, but only part of the data you are searching for is known, then SQL provides the ability to use wildcard characters as part of the search argument.

We wanted to search for Preferred Terms that starts with letter D. By specifying a query using the wildcard character percent sign (%) in a WHERE clause with the LIKE operator, the query results will consist of all rows starts with the letter 'D' as follows.

```
Proc SQL;
        Select Patid, Socterm, Pterm from YLP.Events
        Where Upcase (Pterm) like 'D%';
Quit;
```

If we want to search preferred terms that ends with 'S'

```
Proc SQL;
        Select Patid, Socterm, Pterm from YLP.Events
        Where Upcase (Pterm) like '%S';
Quit;
```

If we want to search preferred terms that has second letter 'A'

```
Proc SQL;
        Select Patid, Socterm, Pterm from YLP.Events
        Where Upcase (Pterm) like '_A%';
Quit;
```

Removing Rows with Duplicate Values:

When the same value is contained in several rows in a table, SQL can remove the rows with duplicate values. By specifying the ***DISTINCT keyword*** prior to the column that is being selected in the SELECT statement automatically removes duplicate rows as illustrated in the following SQL code.

- To select unique values of one or more columns the DISTINCT keyword is used.

```
Proc SQL;
        Select Distinct Pterm as TOTPT from YLP.Events;
Quit;

Proc SQL;
        Select Distinct Socterm from YLP.Events;
Quit;
```

To Count the number of Pterms we use COUNT Clause

```
Proc SQL;
        Select Count (Distinct SOC) as Uniqsoc from YLP.Events;
Quit;
```

Creating Macro Variables by using Proc SQL INTO clause

The PROC SQL SELECT statement is also useful for copying the run time contents of columns into one or more macro variables. The macro variables are each preceded by a colon and all follow the keyword INTO.

```
Proc SQL;
        Select Count (Distinct Patid) from YLP.Demog Where Sex eq 1;
Quit;

Proc SQL;
        Select Count (distinct Patid) INTO: Totfem from YLP.
        Demog
        Where Sex eq 1;
Quit;
```

Check whether the macro variable is created or not

```
        %Put _User_;
```

Joining Tables

Joining tables is a way of bringing rows from different tables together. Rows are usually joined on a key column or columns. If the value of the key(s) in both tables is equal, the rows are joined.

PROC SQL is very useful for joining tables by observation key values. SQL table joins usually execute faster than DATA step Merges, and SQL joins do not require the key columns (BY variables) to be sorted prior to the join. Another important difference between a SQL join and a DATA step Merge is when there are duplicate key values a complete Cartesian product is formed instead of just matching successive observations from each data set. For this reason, 'many to many' SQL joins are valid.

Joins are processed in two distinct phases. The first phase determines whether a FROM clause references two or more tables. When it does, a virtual table, known as the Cartesian product, is created resulting in each row in the first table being combined with each row in the second table, and so forth. The Cartesian product (internal virtual table) can be extremely large since it represents all possible combinations of rows and columns in the joined tables.

The second phase of every join Processes, if present, is specified in the WHERE clause. When a WHERE clause is specified, the number of rows in the Cartesian product is reduced to satisfy this expression. This data Subsetting Process generally results in a more manageable end product containing meaningful data.

Types of Joins

A conceptual view of a join involves combining all rows from the contributing tables and then eliminating those that do not meet the WHERE criteria (equality on the keys).

There are two primary types of joins in SQL, an Equi-join and a Cartesian join.

Cartesian joins: Do not use equality in the WHERE clause or do not use a WHERE clause. This forces each row of the first table to be combined with all rows from the second table if they meet the WHERE criteria.

Equi-joins: Use equality in the WHERE clause. Rows with matching key values are joined. The keys must be of the same length and data type.

Both types of joins allow columns from multiple tables to be included in one where clause. All contributing tables are listed in the FROM clause. Columns with the same names on one or more tables must be qualified by preceding the column name with the name of the contributing table (separated by a period).

Joining more than two tables:

More than two tables can be joined in a single query. A different key can be used to join different tables.

```
Data Events;
Input Patid Aeterm $ @@;
Datalines;
101 Headache 104 Vomit 105 DrySkin
107 Anxiety 108 Backpain 109 Nausea
;
Run;

Data Conmed;
Input Patid Cmname $ @@;
Datalines;
101 Nise 103 Crocin 105 Evion
106 Revital 107 Trika 108 Voveran
;
Run;
```

Creating a Cartesian product:

When a WHERE clause is omitted, all possible combinations of rows from each table is produced. This form of join is known as the Cartesian product.

- If we join two tables with the first table consisting of 5 rows and the second table with 4 rows. The result of these two tables would consist of 20 rows.
- Very rarely is there a need to perform a join operation in SQL where a WHERE clause is not specified.

```
Proc SQL;
        Select * from Events, Conmed;
Quit;
Proc SQL;
        Select * from Events cross join Conmed;
Quit;
```

Concatenation

```
Proc SQL;
        Select * from Events union join Conmed;
Quit;
```

Performing Inner join

An inner join returns a result set for all of the rows in a table that have one or more matching rows in another table, based on the matching criteria (also known as join conditions) that are specified in the ON clause.

```
PROC SQL;
Create Table Both AS
Select * from Events, Conmed
Where Events.Patid=Conmed.Patid;
Quit;

Proc SQL;
Create Table Both AS
Select * from Events inner join Conmed
ON Events. Patid = Conmed. Patid;
Quit;
```

Joins and Table Aliases:

Table aliases provide a 'short-cut' way to reference one or more tables in Joins. One or more aliases are specified so columns can be selected with a minimal number of keystrokes.

The following SQL code illustrates a join on two tables with Patid specified as the connecting column.

```
PROC SQL;
        Create Table Both AS
        Select * from Events as A Inner join Conmed as C
        ON A. Patid = C. Patid;
Quit;
```

The two main points to note are the FROM and the ON clauses. The FROM clause contains both source tables and corresponding aliases, A for Events, and C for Conmed. The keywords INNER JOIN specify the type of join. The ON statement specifies one or more key columns and any related logical operators (In this case =). Column attributes remain unchanged unless they are altered in the SELECT statement.

Performing Outer join

An outer join returns rows that match across tables (as in the inner join) plus non matching rows from one or more tables.

Using Left join

In Left Join all the observations are taken from the Events (A) table and only matching observations from the Conmed (B) table. Columns taken from the B table are substituted with missing values where a key match does not occur.

```
PROC SQL;
        Create Table LJoin AS
        Select * from Events as A Left join Conmed as C
        ON A. Patid = C. Patid;
Quit;
```

Using Right join

A 'right' join considers the key values in the 'right' (B) table first, before performing the matching Process. The following code performs a 'right' join on the same two tables.

```
PROC SQL;
        Create Table RJoin AS
        Select * from Events as A Right join Conmed as C
        ON A. Patid = C. Patid;
Quit;
```

The missing values are where observations are present in Conmed (B) and have no matching observations in Events (A).

Using Full join

Full join is a combination of the 'left' and 'right' joins. A full outer join, specified with the keywords FULL JOIN and ON, selects all matching and non matching rows.

```
PROC SQL;
        Create Table FJoin AS
        Select * from Events as A Full join Conmed as C
        ON A. Patid = C. Patid;
Quit;
```

Joining more than two tables

More than two tables can be joined in a single query. A different key can be used to join different tables.

```
Data Dummy.Events;
Input Patid Aeterm $ @@;
Datalines;
101 Headache 104 Vomit 105 DrySkin
107 Anxiety 108 Backpain 109 Nausea
;
Run;
```

```
Data Dummy.Conmed;
Input Patid Cmname $ @@;
Datalines;
101 Nise 103 Crocin 105 Evion
106 Revital 107 Trika 108 Voveran
;
Run;

Data Dummy.Dose;
Input Patid Cmname $ Dose Doseu $ @@;
Datalines;
101 Nise 100 mg 103 Crocin 500 mg 105 Evion 400 mg
106 Revital . . 107 Trika 0.5 mg 108 Voveran 50 mg
;
Run;

Proc SQL;
        Create Table Detail as
        Select A. Patid, A. Aeterm, C. Cmname, D.dose, D.Doseu
        from Dummy. Events as A, Dummy. Conmed as C,
Dummy. Dose as D
        Where A. Patid = C. Patid and C. Cmname = D.Cmname;
Quit;
```

Reasons for using the SQL Procedure:

- Merging 3 or more data sets without common keys.
- Merging on ranges.
- Summarizing on a calculated value.
- Calculations involving summary values.
- Selecting detail rows based on summary values.
- Less code to understand and maintain by a SAS programmer.
- Non SAS programmers can 'read' SAS programs using the SQL Procedure

Some people want it to happen, some wish it would happen, others make it happen.

Michael Jordan

STEP 13

CDISC SDTM

CDISC: Clinical Data Interchange Standards Consortium is Open, multidisciplinary, non-profit organization with a mission to develop and support global, platform-independent data standards.

- The mission of CDISC is to lead the development of global, vendor-neutral, platform independent standards to improve data quality and accelerate product development in our industry.

CDISC Standards

- Study Data Tabulation Model -- ***SDTM***
- Analysis Dataset Model -- ***ADaM***
- Operational Data Model --***ODM***
- Case Report Tabulation Data Definition Specifications (Define. xml) -- ***CRTDDS***

Introduction:

- SDTM (Study Data Tabulation Model) defines a standard structure for human clinical trial (study) data tabulations that are to be submitted to a regulatory authority such as the United States Food and Drug Administration (FDA).
- Tabulation datasets are electronic listings of individual observations for a subject that comprise the essential data reported from a clinical trial.
- SDTM facilitates data interchange between partners, providers, regulatory authorities.
- The standardized datasets will support the FDA's efforts to develop a repository for all submitted trial data, and a suite of standard review tools to access, manipulate, and view the tabulations.

- These data standards are also expected to benefit industry by streamlining the flow of data from collection through submission.
- SDTM helps to reduce the review and approval time of clinical data submission. Hence, the pharmaceutical companies are able to launch drugs in lesser time. This benefits mankind because of better and quicker control of diseases.

Each variable can be classified according to its Role.

- A Role determines the type of information conveyed by the variable about each distinct observation and how it can be used.

Variables can be classified into four major roles:

Identifier variables, such as those that identify the study, subject, domain, and sequence number of the record.

Topic variables, which specify the focus of the observation (such as the name of a lab test). There is only one per dataset.

Timing variables, which describe the start and end of observation, and/or when it was collected.

Qualifier variables: Describes the attributes and results of the observation. (Such as units and Descriptive adjectives).

The set of Qualifier variables can be further categorized into five sub-classes:

Grouping Qualifiers are used to group together a collection of observations within the same domain. Examples include --CAT and --SCAT.

Result Qualifiers describe the specific results associated with the topic variable in a Findings dataset. They answer the question raised by the topic variable. Result Qualifiers are --ORRES, --STRESC, and --STRESN.

Synonym Qualifiers, specify an alternative name for a particular variable in an observation. Examples include --MODIFY and --DECOD, which are equivalent terms for a --TRT or --TERM topic variable, --TEST and --LOINC which are equivalent terms for a --TESTCD.

Record Qualifiers, define additional attributes of the observation record as a whole (rather than describing a particular variable within a record). Examples include --REASND, AESLIFE, and all other SAE flag variables in the AE domain; AGE, SEX, and RACE in the DM domain; and --BLFL, --POS, --LOC, --SPEC, --LOT, and --NAM in a Findings domain

Variable Qualifiers are used to further modify or describe a specific variable within an observation and are only meaningful in the context of the variable they qualify. Examples include --ORRESU, --ORNRHI, and --ORNRLO, all of which are Variable Qualifiers of --ORRES; and --DOSU, which is a Variable Qualifier of --DOSE.

Let us look at a statement, try to find out the variables in that statement

Subject CT2101 had skin rash a week after the dose of 10mg of study drug XYZ.

- Identifier variable : CT2101
- Topic Variable : Adverse Event term 'skin rash'
- Timing Variable : 1 week= 7 days
- Variable Qualifier : Dose = 10 Dose Unit =mg

SDTM Domains

A domain is defined as a collection of logically related observations with a common topic. Each domain dataset is distinguished by a unique, two-character code that should be used consistently throughout the submission. This code, which is stored in the SDTM variable named DOMAIN, is used as:

- As the dataset name
- The value of the DOMAIN variable in that dataset
- Prefix for most variable names in that dataset.

For e.g. Demographics (Domain which describes the characteristics of the subject such as age, height, weight, sex, country etc) is represented as DM. DM will be stored in SDTM as a dataset name. Prefix for some variable names in that dataset. For E.g. AE is the code for Adverse Event domain. The variable AETERM is derived from AE (domain) and TERM (actual event).

Each row represents the observations recorded for the domain.

- The observations are classified as Intervention class, Event Class or Findings Class.
- Each class contains variables that make up the columns in the domain structure.

- The variables are categorized into different roles (based on the information they contain).

Observations

- Observations can be described by a series of named variables. Each variable normally corresponds to a column in a dataset.
- Most variables in a domain begin with a prescribed prefix.
- An observation can be classified as one of three major types: Interventions, Events, or Findings.

Interventions:

Investigational treatments, therapeutic treatments, and surgical Procedures administered to the subject either as specified by the study protocol (e.g., "***Exposure***"), coincident with the study assessment period (e.g., "***Concomitant Medications***"), or ***self-administered*** by the subject (such as alcohol, tobacco, or caffeine). ***One record per constant dosing /treatment interval.***

Events:

Planned protocol milestones such as randomization and study completion ("disposition"), and occurrences, conditions, or incidents independent of planned study evaluations occurring during the trial (e.g., "adverse events") or prior to the trial (e.g., "medical history"). ***One record per event.***

Findings:

The Findings class captures the observations resulting from planned evaluations (e.g. lab tests, ECGs, microscopic findings), to address specific tests or questions such as laboratory tests, ECG testing, and questions listed on questionnaires. ***One record per finding result or measurement.***

Each observation class has a defined set of standard variables. These standard variables, along with Identifiers and Timing Variables, both of which can be used in all observation classes, are the building blocks for constructing SDTM domains. Variables other than the standard ones for each class must be represented in a ***SUPPQUAL*** dataset.

Generally for any class of observation, the variables are as follows:

Topic: This is exclusive for a particular observation class. It specifies the focus of the observation. E.g. - - TRT is the topic variable for

Intervention Class. For the Exposure domain EX the variable ***EXTRT*** will describe the name of the study drug given to the subject.

Identifier: These identify the study, subject and the sequence number of the record. These are common for all the domains/classes. E.g. ***USUBJID, STUDYID***

Timing: Describe the timings (Start date/time and End date/time). E.g. ***EXSTDTC*** (Start date/ time of study drug).

Qualifier: These describe the results or additional characteristics of the observation. The list of Qualifier variables varies with each observation class. For e.g. ***EXDOSU*** will give the units of the study drug, ***CMROUTE*** will explain the route of administration of the concomitant medicine (CM).

Rule Variable: This expresses an executable method to define the start rule or end rule or looping condition. This variable is meant for the Trial Design Domains (TV, TE).

- All datasets are structured with rows representing observations and columns representing variables.
- Each dataset is described by metadata definitions that provide information about the variables used in the dataset.
- The metadata are described in a data definition document named 'Define' that is submitted with the data to regulatory authorities.
- Data stored in SDTM datasets include both YLP (as originally collected on CRF) and derived values (e.g., converted into standard units, or computed on the basis of multiple values, such as an average).

Define specifies seven distinct metadata attributes to describe SDTM data:

- The Variable Name limited to 8 characters.
- A descriptive Variable Label, using up to 40 characters, which should be unique for each variable in the dataset.
- The data Type (e.g., whether the variable value is a character or numeric)
- The set of controlled terminology for the value or the presentation format of the variable (Controlled Terms or Format)

- The Origin of each variable, such as whether it was collected on a CRF or derived.
- The Role of the variable, which determines how the variable is used in the dataset., Roles are used to represent the categories of variables such as Identifier, Topic, Timing, or the five types of Qualifiers. Since these roles are predefined for all domains that follow the general observation classes, they do not need to be specified by sponsors in their Define data definition document.
- Comments or other relevant information about the variable or its data included by the sponsor as necessary.

Demographics -DM:

This is a standardized set of observations in a specific structure. The Demographics domain describes the essential characteristics of the study subjects, and is used by reviewers for selecting populations for analysis. The values of ARM and ARMCD in DM must match entries in the Trial Arms (TA) dataset E.g. RACE: Asian, Country: USA, Sex: M.

Comments: CO

When collected, comments should be submitted in a single Comments domain. The Comments domain should not include any Identifiers or Timing variables other than those specific for the domain.

The Comments special-purpose domain provides a solution for submitting free-text comments related to data in one or more SDTM domains or collected on a separate CRF page dedicated to comments

Exposure: EX

This domain records the details of the subject's exposure to protocol-specified study treatment. Study treatment is defined as any intervention that is defined as a test material and is usually but need not necessarily be applied to a subject. EXCAT and EXSCAT may be used when appropriate to categorize treatments into categories and subcategories. EXTRT captures the name of the investigational treatment and it is the topic variable. EXTRT should only include the treatment name and should not include dosage, formulation or other quallfying information.

E.g.: EXTRT: STUDYDRUG, DOSADM: 20, EXDOSADMU: mg, EXDOSFRM: Tablet.

Adverse Event: AE

Adverse Event domain captures the adverse events during the course of the clinical trial. An adverse event is an unanticipated negative effect associated with the use of experimental drugs, devices or Procedures that is serious or unexpected and possibly related to the trial.

AETERM captures the verbatim term collected for the event. It is the topic variable for the AE dataset. AEDECOD is the preferred term derived by the sponsor from the coding dictionary.

E.g. AETERM: Anorexia, AECAT: General, AESER: N

Disposition: DS

The Disposition dataset provides an accounting for all subjects who entered the study and may include protocol milestones, such as randomization, as well as the subject's completion status or reason for discontinuation for the entire study or each phase or segment of the study, including screening and post-treatment follow up.

The controlled terminology will depend on the value of DSCAT. When DSCAT = "DISPOSITION EVENT", DSTERM contains either "COMPLETE" or, If the subject did not complete, specific verbatim information about the disposition event.

When DSCAT="PROTOCOL MILESTONE", DSTERM and DSDECOD will contain the same value drawn from the sponsor's controlled terminology. E.g. DSTERM: Disease Progression, DSDECOD: PROGRESSIVE DISEASE, DSCAT: Disposition Event

Substance Use: SU

To capture the substance use information that may be used to assess the efficacy and/or safety of therapies that look to mitigate the effects of chronic substance use. SUTRT captures the verbatim or the pre specified text collected for the substance. It is a required variable.

E.g. SUTRT: Cigarettes, SUDOSU: Pack, SUDOSFRQ: Per Day.

Medical History: MH

This domain Includes subject's prior and concomitant ***conditions*** at start of the Trial. Information includes general medical history and gynecological history. MHTERM captures the verbatim term collected for the condition or event. MHTERM is the topic variable for MH dataset.

MHENRF is used when the relative timing assessment is coincident with the start of the study reference period for subjects represented in Demographics dataset. (RFSTDTC).

E.g. MHTERM: Angina Pectoris, MHDICT: MedDRA

Concomitant Medication: CM

Domain contains the information related to Concomitant Medications or Therapies given on an as needed basis and the usual background medication or therapies given for a condition.

CMTRT should only include the medication/therapy name and should not include dosage, formulation, or other qualifying information.

E.g. CMTRT: Paracetamol, CMDOS: 250, CMDOSU: mg, CMCAT: General.

Protocol Deviations: DV

This model captures the protocol deviations that occurred during the study. These deviations are other than the violated inclusion/exclusion criteria. E.g. Drug XXXX administered during study treatment period.

Clinical Events: CE

This domain captures clinical events of interest that would not be captured as adverse events. The data could be data about the episodes of symptoms of the disease under study. This event could be pre specified on CRF. E.g. Rash, Nausea

ECG Results: EG

CRF data that captures interval measurements and summary information. EGNRIND: can be added to indicate where a result falls with respect to reference range defined by EGORNRLO(EG Original Normal low) and EGORNRHI The Qualifiers: --MODIFY, --BODSYS, --SPEC are not used. e.g. EGTEST: Ventricular Rate, EGPOS: Supine, EGORRES: Abnormal.

Laboratory Test Results: LB

This domain captures laboratory data collected on the CRF or received from the central provider. Value derived by a central lab according to their Procedure is considered rather than derived. For lab test that do not have continuous numeric results, LBSTNRC is populated.

E.g. LBTEST: Glucose, LBCAT: Urine, LBORRESU: mg/dL

Physical Examination: PE

Information about which body systems were examined and specific abnormalities collected. The results are recorded as PEORRES is coded.

E.g. PETESTCD: Head, PELOC: Face, PESTRESC: Normal.

Questionnaires: QS

Questionnaires are analyzed by applying a numeric scoring system to question responses. Questionnaire data may include, but are not limited to subject reported outcomes and validated or non-validated questionnaires. The QS domain is not intended for use in submitting a set of questions grouped on the CRF for convenience of data capture.

E.g. ***QSTEST:*** Healthy as anybody, ***QSSCAT:*** General Health, ***QSORRES:*** True

Subject Characteristics: SC

Subject Characteristics is for data not collected in other domains that are subject-related. Examples: subject initials, eye color, childbearing status, etc. The structure of subject characteristics is based on the Findings general observation class and is an extension of the demographics data. SC contains data that is either not normally expected to change during the trial or whose change is not of interest after the initial collection.

E.g. ***SCTEST:*** Eye Color, ***SCORRES:*** Brown, SCTESTCD: EYECD

Vital Signs: VS

CRF captures measurements such as blood pressure, height, weight, pulse, and body temperature, or derived data such as body mass index. In cases where the LOINC dictionary is used for Vital Sign tests, the permissible variable VSLOINC could be used. VSNRIND can be used to indicate where a result falls with respect to reference range defined by VSORNRLO and VSORNRHI.

E.g. ***VSTEST:*** Systolic Blood Pressure, ***VSPOS:*** Sitting, ***VSORRES***: 154, ***VSSORRESU***: mmHg.

The domains are captured on a case report form.

The Case Report form is annotated with the corresponding variables for the respective domains, for e.g. The initials of the subject would be annotated as SUBJID. The Study Number will be annotated as STUDYID. A combination of the STUDYID and the SUBJID could be annotated as a USUBJID.

SDTM Dates: Represented in ISO 8601 format as a complete date/time, a partial date/time, or an incomplete date/time i.e. YYYY-MM-DDThh:mm:ss

E.g. December 15, 2003 13:15:17 → 2003-12-15T13:15:17

Note: Spaces Are Not Allowed In Any Iso 8601 Representations

DM Domain Specifications:

DOMAIN: *DM*
Description: *Demographics*
Class: *Special Purpose*
Structure: *One record per subject*
Purpose: *Tabulation*
Keys: *STUDYID USUBJID*
Location: *dm.xpt*

Source Datasets: *YLP.DEMOG, YLP.EOS, YLP.SDYTRT, YLP.EVENTS, YLP.SFL, YLP.INVHIST, YLP.RAND.*

Name	***Label***	***Type***	***Origin***	***Comment***	***Core***	***Role***
STUDYID	Study Identifier	Text	Protocol	STUDYID = "**CT10375"**	Req	Identifier
DOMAIN	Domain Abbreviation	Text	Assigned	DOMAIN = "DM"	Req	Identifier
USUBJID	Unique Subject Identifier	Text	Derived	STUDYID ||'-'SUBJID	Req	Identifier
SUBJID	Subject Identifier for the Study	Text	CRF	SUBJID = concatenate DEMOG.SITE and DEMOG.PATID with a "-"	Req	Topic
RFSTDTC	Subject Reference Start Date/ Time	Text	CRF	RFSTDTC = SDYTRT.SDYDOSEDT when VISIT = 3. Use date in ISO format.	Exp	Record Qualifier

RFENDTC	Subject Reference End Date/Time	Text	CRF	RFENDTC = EOS.SDYDOSEDT. Use date in ISO format.	Exp	Record Qualifier
RFXSTDTC	Date/Time of First Study Treatment	Text	Derived	RFXSTDTC = DOSEADM.SDYDOSEDT when VISIT = 3. Use date in ISO format.	Exp	Timing
RFXENDTC	Date/Time of Last Study Treatment	Text	Derived	RFXENDTC = RFENDTC	Exp	Timing
RFICDTC	Date/Time of Informed Consent	Text	CRF Page 3	RFICDTC = DEMOG.ICDT. Use date in ISO format.	Exp	Timing
RFPENDTC	Date/Time of End of Participation	Text	Derived	If not missing EVENTS. DEATHDT Then RFPENDTC = EVENTS. DEATHDT. Use date in ISO format.	Exp	Timing
DTHDTC	Date/Time of Death	Text	CRF	DTHDTC = EVENTS.DEATHDT. Use date in ISO format.	Exp	Timing
DTHFL	Subject Death Flag	Text	Derived	EVENTS.AEOUT = 5 Then DTHFL = "Y"; Otherwise DTHFL = Null	Exp	Timing

SITEID	Study Site Identifier	Text	CRF	For subjects from YLP.SFL Then
				SITEID = SFL.SITE;
				For all other subject Then
				SITEID = DEMOG.SITE
					Req	Record Qualifier

INVID	Investigator Identifier	Text		INVHIST.PI_ID	Perm	Record Qualifier
INVNAM	Investigator Name	Text		INVHIST.PI_NAME	Perm	Synonym Qualifier
BRTHDTC	Date/Time of Birth	Text	CRF	BRTHDTC = DEMOG.BIRTHDT	Perm	Record Qualifier
AGE	Age	Integer	Derived	Consider DEMOG.BIRTHDT and DEMOG. CONDT for subjects from YLP.DEMOG for age calculation	Exp	Record Qualifier
AGEU	Age Units	Text	Assigned	"YEARS"	Exp	Variable Qualifier
SEX	Sex	Text	CRF	For subjects from YLP.SFL: If SFL.SEX = 1 Then SEX = "F"; If SFL.SEX = 2 Then SEX = "M"; For subjects from YLP.DEMOG: If DEMOG.SEX = 1 Then SEX = "F"; If DEMOG.SEX = 2 Then SEX = "M"	Req	Record Qualifier
RACE	Race	Text	Derived, CRF Page 3, 14	***Derivation:*** ""= "MULTIPLE" If more than one value of 1 is populated in DEMOG. RACE1, DEMOG. RACE2, DEMOG. RACE3, DEMOG. RACE4, DEMOG. RACE5;	Exp	Record Qualifier

				"= "MULTIPLE" If more than one value of 1 is populated in SFL. RACE1, SFL. RACE2, SFL. RACE3, SFL. RACE4, SFL. RACE5; or If not more than 1 race is checked Then If DEMOG. RACE = 1 or SFL.RACE = 1 Then RACE = "AMERICAN INDIAN OR ALASKA NATIVE"; If DEMOG. RACE = 2 or SFL.RACE = 2 Then RACE = "ASIAN"; If DEMOG.RACE = 3 or SFL.RACE = 3 Then RACE = "BLACK OR AFRICAN AMERICAN"; If DEMOG.RACE = 4 or SFL.RACE = 4 Then RACE = "NATIVE HAWAIIAN OR OTHER PACIFIC ISLANDER"; If DEMOG.RACE = 5 or SFL.RACE = 5 Then RACE = "WHITE";		
ETHNIC	Ethnicity	Text	CRF	If DEMOG. ETHNIC = 1 Then ETHNIC = "HISPANIC OR LATINO" ; If DEMOG. ETHNIC = 2 Then ETHNIC = "NOT HISPANIC OR LATINO"	Perm	Record Qualifier

ARMCD	Planned Arm Code	Text	Derived	Values for ARMCD: If RAND.TRTCD = 1 Then ARMCD = "PLB" Else If RAND.TRTCD = 2 Then ARMCD = "TD_1MG" Else If RAND.TRTCD = 3 Then ARMCD = "TD_3MG " Else If RAND. TRTCD = 4 Then ARMCD = "TD_6MG" Else If subject is retrieved from YLP.SFL Then ARMCD = "SCRNFAIL" Else ARMCD = "NOTASSGN".	Req	Record Qualifier

ARM	Description of Planned Arm	Text	Derived	Values for ARM: “Placebo” when ARMCD = “PLB” “Test Drug 1 mg” when ARMCD = “TD_1MG” “Test Drug 3 mg” when ARMCD = “TD_3MG” “Test Drug 6 mg” when ARMCD = “TD_6MG” “Screen Failure” when ARMCD = “SCRNFAIL” “Not Assigned” when ARMCD = “NOTASSGN”	Req	Synonym Qualifier
ACTARMCD	Actual Arm Code	Text	Derived	Values for ACTARMCD: If RAND.TRTCD = 1 Then ARMCD = “PLB” Else If RAND.TRTCD = 2 Then ARMCD = “TD_1MG” ElseIf RAND.TRTCD = 3 Then ARMCD = “TD_3MG “ Else If RAND. TRTCD = 4 Then ARMCD = “TD_6MG” Else If subject is retrieved from SDB.	Req	Timing

				SFL Then ARMCD = "SCRNFAIL" Else ARMCD = "NOTASSGN".		
ACTARM	Description of Actual Arm	Text	Derived	Values for ACTARM: "Placebo" when ARMCD = "PLB" "Test Drug 1 mg" when ARMCD = "TD_1MG" "Test Drug 3 mg" when ARMCD = "TD_3MG" "Test Drug 6 mg" when ARMCD = "TD_6MG" "Screen Failure" when ARMCD = "SCRNFAIL" "Not Assigned" when ARMCD = "NOTASSGN"	Req	Timing
COUNTRY	Country	Text	Assigned	If data from YLP.DEMOG Then: If DEMOG.COUNTRY = "US" Then COUNTRY = "USA".	Req	Record Qualifier
DMDTC	Date/Time of Collection	Text	CRF Page 6	DMDTC = DEMOG.VISDT. Use date in ISO format.	Perm	Timing
DMDY	Study Day of Collection	Integer	Derived	Use STUDY DAY calculation concept.	Perm	Timing

CM Domain:

Dataset : CM

Description: Concomitant Medications

Class : Interventions

Structure : One record per medication intervention episode per subject

Purpose : Tabulation

Keys : STUDYID USUBJID CMSTDTC CMCAT CMTRT

Location : cm.xpt

Source Datasets: YLP.CONMED, SDTM.DM

Variable Name	Variable Label	Type	Origin	Data Map	Core	Role
STUDYID	Study Identifier	Text	Protocol	STUDYID = "WHYEL08"	Req	Identifier
DOMAIN	Domain Abbreviation	Text	Assigned	DOMAIN = "CM"	Req	Identifier
USUBJID	Unique Subject Identifier	Text	Derived	STUDYID||'-'|| SUBJID	Req	Identifier
CMSEQ	Sequence Number	Integer	Derived	Derived based on key variables	Req	Identifier
CMGRPID	Group ID	Text	Derived		Perm	Identifier
CMSPID	Sponsor-Defined Identifier	Text	CRF		Perm	Identifier

CMTRT	Reported Name of Drug, Med, or Therapy	Text	CRF	If data from YLP.CONMED Then CMTRT = CONMED.MEDVT;	Req	Topic
CMMODIFY	Modified Reported Name	Text	Assigned		Perm	Synonym Qualifier
CMDECOD	Standardized Medication Name	Text	Assigned	CMDECOD = CONMED. PREFNAM;	Perm	Synonym Qualifier
CMCAT	Category for Medication	Text	CRF	If data from YLP.CONMED and CONMED.MEDTYP = 1 Then CMCAT = "PRIOR"; If data from YLP.CONMED and CONMED.MEDTYP = 2 Then CMCAT = "CONCOMITANT";	Perm	Grouping Qualifier
CMSCAT	Subcategory for Medication	Text	CRF		Perm	Grouping Qualifier
CMPRESP	CM Pre-Specified	Text	Derived		Perm	Record Qualifier
CMOCCUR	CM Occurrence	Text	CRF		Perm	Record Qualifier
CMSTAT	Completion Status	Text	CRF		Perm	Record Qualifier
CMREASND	Reason Medication Not Collected	Text	CRF		Perm	Record Qualifier
CMINDC	Indication	Text	CRF		Perm	Record Qualifier

CMCLAS	Medication Class	Text	Assigned		Perm	Variable Qualifier
CMCLASCD	Medication Class Code	Text	Assigned		Perm	Variable Qualifier
CMDOSE	Dose per Administration	Float	CRF	If data from YLP.CONMED and numeric Then CMDOSE = CONMED.DOSE;	Perm	Record Qualifier
CMDOSTXT	Dose Description	Text		If data from YLP.CONMED and CONMED.DOSE is not map able to CMDOSE Then CMDOSTXT = CONMED.	Perm	Record Qualifier
				DOSE; Example: 15-20, 2 tsp, 2 sprays; If data from YLP.CONMED and CONMED.UNIT is not map able to CMDOSE Then CMDOSTXT = CONMED.UNIT; If data from YLP.CONMED and CONMED.FREQ is not map able to CMDOSE Then CMDOSTXT = CONMED.FREQ; If all 3 Variables can't be mapped Then concatenate all 3. If only CMDOSE and UNIT for example can't be mapped Then map those 2 and populate FREQ in CMDOSFRQ with standard value.		

CMDOSU	Dose Units	Text	CRF	If data from YLP.CONMED Then CMDOSU = CONMED.UNIT; Apply standard Terminology	Perm	Variable Qualifier
CMDOSFRM	Dose Form	Text	CRF		Perm	Record Qualifier
CMDOSFRQ	Dosing Frequency per Interval	Text	CRF	If data from YLP.CONMED Then CMDOSFRQ = CONMED.FREQ; Apply standard Terminology.	Perm	Variable Qualifier
CMDOSTOT	Total Daily Dose	Float	Derived		Perm	Record Qualifier
CMDOSRGM	Intended Dose Regimen	Text	CRF		Perm	Variable Qualifier
CMROUTE	Route of Administration	Text	CRF	If data from YLP.CONMED Then CMROUTE = CONMED.ROUTE; Apply standard Terminology. Check data after each transfer and update spec;	Perm	Variable Qualifier
CMSTDTC	Start Date/Time of Medication	Text	CRF	If data from YLP.CONMED and CONMED.MEDTYP = 1 Then CMSTDTC = null; If data from YLP.CONMED and CONMED.MEDTYP = 2 Then Concatenate CONMED.MSDTD, CONMED.MSDTM and CONMED.MSDTY Check for Partial Dates.	Perm	Timing

CMENDTC	End Date/Time of Medication	Text	CRF	If data from YLP.CONMED Then Concatenate CONMED.MEDTD, CONMED.MEDTM and CONMED.MEDTY Check for Partial Dates Use date in ISO format	Perm	Timing
CMSTDY	Study Day of Start of Medication	Integer	Derived	Use CMSTDTC and RFSTDTC for calculation.	Perm	Timing
CMENDY	Study Day of End of Medication	Integer	Derived	Use CMENDTC and RFENDTC for calculation.	Perm	Timing
CMDUR	Duration of Medication	Text	CRF		Perm	Timing
CMSTRF	Start Relative to Reference Period	Text	CRF		Perm	Timing
CMENRF	End Relative to Reference Period	Text	CRF		Perm	Timing
CMSTRTPT	Start Relative to Reference Time Point	Text	CRF		Perm	Timing
CMSTTPT	Start Reference Time Point	Text	Derived		Perm	Timing
CMENRTPT	End Relative to Reference Time Point	Text	CRF	If data from YLP.CONMED and CONMED.MEDTYP = 2 and CONMED.CMONGO = 1 Then CMENRTPT = “ONGOING”;	Perm	Timing

CMENTPT	End Reference Time Point	Text	CRF	If data from YLP.CONMED and CONMED.MEDTYP = 2 and CONMED.CMONGO = 1 Then CMENTPT = "STUDY END";	Perm	Timing
EPOCH	Epoch	Text	Protocol		Req	Timing
ETCD	Element Code	Text	Assigned		Req	Topic
ELEMENT	Description of Element	Text	Protocol		Req	Synonym Qualifier

AE Domain

DOMAIN : AE
Description : Adverse Events
Class : Events
Structure : One record per adverse event per subject
Purpose : Tabulation
Keys : STUDYID USUBJID AESTDTC AEDECOD AETERM
Location : ae.xpt
Source Datasets : *YLP.EVENTS, SDTM.DM*

<table>
<tr><th>Variable Name</th><th>Variable Label</th><th>Type</th><th>Origin</th><th>Comment</th><th>Core</th><th>Role</th></tr>
<tr><td>STUDYID</td><td>Study Identifier</td><td>Text</td><td>Protocol</td><td>STUDYID = “WHYEL08”</td><td>Req</td><td>Identifier</td></tr>
<tr><td>DOMAIN</td><td>Domain Abbreviation</td><td>Text</td><td>Assigned</td><td>DOMAIN = “AE”</td><td>Req</td><td>Identifier</td></tr>
<tr><td>USUBJID</td><td>Unique Subject Identifier</td><td>Text</td><td>Derived</td><td>STUDYID||’-‘|| SUBJID</td><td>Req</td><td>Identifier</td></tr>
<tr><td>AESEQ</td><td>Sequence Number</td><td>Integer</td><td>Derived</td><td>Derived based on key variables</td><td>Req</td><td>Identifier</td></tr>
<tr><td>AEGRPID</td><td>Group ID</td><td>Text</td><td>Derived</td><td></td><td>Perm</td><td>Identifier</td></tr>
</table>

AEREFID	Reference ID	Text	CRF		Perm	Identifier
AESPID	Sponsor-Defined Identifier	Text	Assigned	AESPID = EVENTS.AESEQ. This variable should be in Z2. Format.	Perm	Identifier
AETERM	Reported Term for the Adverse Event	Text	CRF	AETERM = EVENTS.AEVT	Req	Topic
AEMODIFY	ModIfied Reported Term	Text	Assigned		Perm	Synonym Qualifier
AELLT	Lowest Level Term	Text	Assigned	AELLT = EVENTS.LLT_NAME	Exp	Record Qualifier
AELLTCD	Lowest Level Term Code	Integer	Assigned	AELLTCD = EVENTS.LLT_CODE	Exp	Record Qualifier
AEDECOD	Dictionary-Derived Term	Text	Assigned	AEDECOD = EVENTS.PT_NAME	Req	Synonym Qualifier
AEPTCD	Preferred Term Code	Integer	Assigned	AEPTCD = EVENTS.PT_CODE	Exp	Record Qualifier
AEHLT	High Level Term	Text	Assigned	AEHLT = EVENTS.HLT_NAME	Exp	Record Qualifier
AEHLTCD	High Level Term Code	Integer	Assigned	AEHLTCD = EVENTS.HLT_CODE	Exp	Record Qualifier
AEHLGT	High Level Group Term	Text	Assigned		Exp	Record Qualifier
AEHLGTCD	High Level Group Term Code	Integer	Assigned		Exp	Record Qualifier

AECAT	Category for Adverse Event	Text	CRF	If EVENTS.AETYPE = 1 Then AECAT = "Pretreatment Event"; If EVENTS.AETYPE = 2 Then AECAT = "Adverse Event"	Perm	Grouping Qualifier
AESCAT	Subcategory for Adverse Event	Text	CRF		Perm	Grouping Qualifier
AEPRESP	Pre-Specified Adverse Event	Text	Derived		Perm	Record Qualifier
AEBODSYS	Body System or Organ Class	Text	Assigned	AEBODSYS = EVENTS.SOC_NAME	Exp	Record Qualifier
AEBDSYCD	Body System or Organ Class Code	Integer	Assigned	AEBDSYCD = EVENTS.SOC_CODE	Exp	Record Qualifier
AESOC	Primary System Organ Class	Text	Assigned	AESOC = EVENTS.SOC_NAME	Exp	Record Qualifier
AESOCCD	Primary System Organ Class Code	Integer	Assigned	AESOC = EVENTS.SOC_CODE	Exp	Record Qualifier
AELOC	Location of Event	Text	CRF		Perm	Record Qualifier
AESEV	Severity/Intensity	Text	CRF	If EVENTS.AEINTE = 1 Then AESEV = "MILD"; If EVENTS.AEINTE = 2 Then AESEV = "MODERATE"; If EVENTS.AEINTE = 3 Then AESEV = "SEVERE"	Perm	Record Qualifier

AESER	Serious Event	Text	CRF	If EVENTS.AESER = 1 Then AESER = "Y"; If EVENTS.AESER = 2 Then AESER = "N"	Exp	Record Qualifier
AEACN	Action Taken with Study Treatment	Text	CRF	If EVENTS.AEACT = 1 Then AEACN = "DRUG WITHDYLPN"; If EVENTS.AEACT = 2 Then AEACN = "DOSE NOT CHANGED"; If EVENTS.AEACT = 3 Then AEACN = "UNKNOWN";		
				If EVENTS.AEACT = 4 Then AEACN = "NOT APPLICABLE"; If EVENTS.AEACT = 5 Then AEACN = "DOSE REDUCED"; If EVENTS.AEACT = 6 Then AEACN = "DOSE INCREASED"; If EVENTS.AEACT = 7 Then AEACN = "DRUG INTERRUPTED"	Exp	Record Qualifier
AEACNOTH	Other Action Taken	Text	CRF		Perm	Record Qualifier
AEREL	Causality	Text	CRF	If EVENTS.AERELAN= 1 Then AEREL = "Y"; If EVENTS.AERELAN= 2 Then AEREL = "N"	Exp	Record Qualifier
AERELNST	Relationship to Non-Study Treatment	Text	CRF		Perm	Record Qualifier

AEPATT	Pattern of Adverse Event	Text	CRF	If EVENTS.AEFREQ = 1 Then AEPATT = "Intermittent"; If EVENTS.AEFREQ = 2 Then AEPATT = "Continuous"	Perm	Record Qualifier
AEOUT	Outcome of Adverse Event	Text	CRF	If EVENTS.AEOUT = 1 Then AEOUT = "RECOVERED /RESOLVED"; If EVENTS.AEOUT = 2 Then AEOUT = "RECOVERING/ RESOLVING"; If EVENTS.AEOUT = 3 Then AEOUT = "NOT RECOVERED /NOT RESOLVED"; If EVENTS.AEOUT = 4 Then AEOUT = "RECOVERED /RESOLVED WITH SEQUELAE"; If EVENTS.AEOUT = 5 Then AEOUT = "FATAL"; If EVENTS.AEOUT = 6 Then AEOUT = "UNKNOWN"	Perm	Record Qualifier
AESCAN	Involves Cancer	Text	CRF		Perm	Record Qualifier
AESCONG	Congenital Anomaly or Birth Defect	Text	CRF		Perm	Record Qualifier
AESDISAB	Persistent or Significant Disability/Incapacity	Text	CRF		Perm	Record Qualifier
AESDTH	Results in Death	Text	CRF		Perm	Record Qualifier

AESHOSP	Requires or Prolongs Hospitalization	Text	CRF		Perm	Record Qualifier
AESLIFE	Is Life Threatening	Text	CRF		Perm	Record Qualifier
AESOD	Occurred with Overdose	Text	CRF		Perm	Record Qualifier
AESMIE	Other Medically Important Serious Event	Text	CRF		Perm	Record Qualifier
AECONTRT	Concomitant or Additional Trt Given	Text	CRF		Perm	Record Qualifier
AETOXGR	Standard Toxicity Grade	Text	CRF		Perm	Record Qualifier
AESTDTC	Start Date/Time of Adverse Event	Text	CRF	Concatenate EVENTS. AESTDT and EVENTS. AESTTM convert it to an ISO format.	Exp	Timing
AEENDTC	End Date/Time of Adverse Event	Text	CRF	Concatenate EVENTS.AEENDT and EVENTS. AEENTM convert it to an ISO format.	Exp	Timing
AESTDY	Study Day of Start of Adverse Event	Integer	Derived	Use AESTDTC, RFSTDTC for calculation.	Perm	Timing
AEENDY	Study Day of End of Adverse Event	Integer	Derived	Use AEENDTC, RFENDTC for calculation.	Perm	Timing
AEDUR	Duration of Adverse Event	Text	CRF		Perm	Timing

AEENRF	End Relative to Reference Period	Text	CRF		Perm	Timing
AEENRTPT	End Relative to Reference Time Point	Text	CRF	If EVENTS.AEONGO = 1 Then AEENRTPT = "ONGOING"	Perm	Timing
AEENTPT	End Reference Time Point	Text	CRF	If EVENTS.AEONGO = 1 Then AEENTPT = "STUDY END"	Perm	Timing
EPOCH	Epoch	Text	Protocol		Req	Timing
ETCD	Element Code	Text	Assigned		Req	Topic
ELEMENT	Description of Element	Text	Protocol		Req	Synonym Qualifier

LB Domain:

Dataset : *LB*
Description : *Laboratory Test Results*
Class : *Findings*
Structure : *One record per lab test per time point per visit per subject*
Purpose : *Tabulation*
Keys : *STUDYID USUBJID LBCAT LBTESTCD LBDTC VISITNUM LBTPTNUM LBREFID*
Source : *YLP.CLILAB, YLP.OGTT, YLP.GLU, YLP.LAB, YLP.PT, SDTM.TV, SDTM.DM*

Variable Name	Variable Label	Type	Origin	Comment	Core	Role
STUDYID	Study Identifier	Text	Protocol	STUDYID = “WHYEL08”	Req	Identifier
DOMAIN	Domain Abbreviation	Text	Assigned	DOMAIN = “LB”	Req	Identifier
USUBJID	Unique Subject Identifier	Text	Derived		Req	Identifier
LBSEQ	Sequence Number	Integer	Derived		Req	Identifier
LBGRPID	Group ID	Text	Derived		Perm	Identifier
LBREFID	Specimen ID	Text	CRF	Values for LBREFID when data comes from YLP. LAB: LBREFID = LAB.LBREFID	Perm	Identifier

LBSPID	Sponsor-Defined Identifier	Text	Assigned		Perm	Identifier
LBTESTCD	Lab Test or Examination Short Name	Text	Assigned, CRF	Values for LBTESTCD when data comes from YLP. LAB: LBTESTCD = LAB.LBTEST	Req	Topic
LBTEST	Lab Test or Examination Name	Text	Assigned	Values for LBTEST when data comes from YLP.LAB. LBTEST = LAB.LTSTNAM Values for LBTEST	Req	Synonym Qualifier
LBCAT	Category for Lab Test	Text	Assigned	Values for LBCAT: Merge with external file specified in “General Information Tab” to obtain LBCAT, use column “Reporting Category” For analyte with no category in the repository, map using the Supplemental Lab Cat information.	Exp	Grouping Qualifier
LBSCAT	Subcategory for Lab Test	Text			Perm	Grouping Qualifier
LBORRES	Result or Finding in Original Units	Text	CRF	Values for LBORRES when data comes from YLP. LAB: LBORRES = LAB.LBORRESC or LBORRES = LAB.LBORRESN	Exp	Result Qualifier

LBORRESU	Original Units	Text	CRF	Values for LBORRESU when data comes from YLP. LAB: LBORRESU = LAB.LBORRESU	Exp	Variable Qualifier
LBORNRLO	Reference Range Lower Limit in Original Unit	Text	Derived	Values for LBORNRLO when data comes from YLP. LAB: LBORNRLO = LAB.LBORNRLO	Exp	Variable Qualifier
LBORNRHI	Reference Range Upper Limit in Original Unit	Text	Derived	Values for LBORNRHI when data comes from YLP. LAB: LBORNRHI = LAB.LBORNRHI	Exp	Variable Qualifier
LBSTRESC	Character Result/ Finding in Standard Format	Text	Derived	Values for LBSTRESC: LBSTRESC is derived from LBORRES by using the CV to SI conversion factors provided in the lab repository.	Exp	Result Qualifier
LBSTRESN	Numeric Result/ Finding in Standard Units	Float	Derived	Values for LBSTRESN: LBSTRESC is derived from LBORRES by using the CV to SI conversion factors provided in the lab repository.	Exp	Result Qualifier
LBSTRESU	Standard Units	Text	Derived	Values for LBSTRESU: LBSTRESC is based on the units provided in the lab repository for SI results.	Exp	Variable Qualifier
LBSTNRLO	Reference Range Lower Limit-Std Units	Float		Values for LBSTNRLO: LBSTNRLO is derived from LBORRES by using the CV to SI conversion factors provided in the lab repository.	Exp	Variable Qualifier

LBSTNRHI	Reference Range Upper Limit-Std Units	Float		Values for LBSTNRHI: LBSTNRHI is derived from LBORRES by using the CV to SI conversion factors provided in the lab repository.	Exp	Variable Qualifier
LBSTNRC	Reference Range for Char Result Std Units	Text		Values for LBSTNRC when data comes from YLP.LAB: LBSTNRC = LAB.LBORNRC	Perm	Variable Qualifier
LBNRIND	Reference Range Indicator	Text		Values for LBNRIND when data comes from YLP.LAB: LBNRIND = "LOW" when LAB.AFLAGO = "L" LBNRIND = "" when LAB.AFLAGO = "" LBNRIND = "HIGH" when LAB.AFLAGO = "H"	Exp	Variable Qualifier
LBSTAT	Completion Status	Text	CRF	Values for LBSTAT when data comes from YLP.LAB: LBSTAT = LAB.LBSTAT Values for LBSTAT when data comes from YLP.OGTT: LBSTAT = "NOT DONE" when OGTT.OGTTQ = 2 Values for LBSTAT when data comes from YLP.CLILAB: LBSTAT = "NOT DONE" when CLILAB.BLOQ = 2 and LBCAT = "BIOCHEMISTRY" LBSTAT = "NOT DONE" when CLILAB.URIQ = 2 and LBCAT = "URINALYSIS" Values for LBSTAT when data comes from YLP.PT: LBSTAT = "NOT DONE" when PT.PTRLT = 4;	Perm	Record Qualifier

LBREASND	Reason Test Not Done	Text	CRF	Values for LBREASND when data comes from YLP.LAB: LBREASND = LAB.LBREASND when LBSTAT = "NOT DONE" Values for LBREASND when data comes from YLP,CLILAB: LBREASND = CLILAB.BSPY when LBSTAT = "NOT DONE" and LBCAT = "CHEMISTRY" LBREASND = CLILAB.USPY when LBSTAT = "NOT DONE" and LBCAT = "URINALYSIS"	Perm	Record Qualifier
LBNAM	Vendor Name	Text	External file	Values for LBNAM when data comes from YLP.LAB:	Perm	Record Qualifier
LBLOINC	LOINC Code	Text	External file		Perm	Synonym Qualifier
LBSPEC	Specimen Type	Text	External file	Value for LBSPEC when data comes from YLP.LAB: LBSPEC = "BLOOD" when LAB.LBSPEC = 1, LBSPEC = "PLASMA" when LAB.LBSPEC = 2, LBSPEC = "SERUM" when LAB.LBSPEC = 3, LBSPEC = "URINE" when LAB.LBSPEC = 4, LBSPEC = "STOOL" when LAB.LBSPEC = 5.	Perm	Record Qualifier
LBSPCCND	Specimen Condition	Text	External file		Perm	Record Qualifier
LBMETHOD	Method of Test or Examination	Text	External file	Values for LBMETHOD when data comes from YLP.LAB: LBMETHOD = LAB.LBMETHOD	Perm	Record Qualifier

LBBLFL	Baseline Flag	Text	Derived	Baseline flag should correspond to the last available non-missing value on or before the date of the first dose of study drug, where OGTTYN is not "Y" and the time point is not populated.	Exp	Record Qualifier
LBFAST	Fasting Status	Text	External file	Values for LBFAST when data comes from YLP.LAB: LBFAST = LAB.FAST	Perm	Record Qualifier
LBDRVFL	Derived Flag	Text	Derived		Perm	Record Qualifier
LBTOX	Toxicity	Text	Assigned		Perm	Variable Qualifier
LBTOXGR	Standard Toxicity Grade	Text	Derived		Perm	Variable Qualifier
VISITNUM	Visit Number	Integer	Assigned	Values for VISITNUM when data comes from YLP. LAB: VISITNUM = LAB.VISIT	Exp	Timing
VISIT	Visit Name	Text	Assigned	Assign VISIT as defined in SDTM.TV by merging on VISITNUM.	Perm	Timing
VISITDY	Planned Study Day of Visit	Integer	Assigned	Assign VISITDY as defined in SDTM.TV by merging on VISITNUM.	Perm	Timing
LBDTC	Date/Time of Specimen Collection	Text	CRF	Value for LBDTC when data comes from YLP.LAB: LBDTC = LAB.SAMPDT and LAB.SAMPTM. Use date in ISO format.	Exp	Timing

LBENDTC	End Date/Time of Specimen Collection	Text	CRF		Perm	Timing
LBDY	Study Day of Specimen Collection	Integer	Derived		Perm	Timing
LBTPT	Planned Time Point Name	Text	CRF	data comes from YLP.LAB: LBTPT = “-10” when LAB.TPTNUM = -10” LBTPT = “30” when LAB.TPTNUM = “30” LBTPT = “60” when LAB.TPTNUM = “60” LBTPT = “90” when LAB.TPTNUM = “90” LBTPT = “120” when LAB.TPTNUM = 120”	Perm	Timing
LBTPTNUM	Planned Time Point Number	Integer	Derived	data comes from YLP.LAB: If TPTNUM eq “-10” Then LBTPTNUM = 1, If TPTNUM eq “30” Then LBTPTNUM = 2, If TPTNUM eq “60” Then LBTPTNUM = 3, If TPTNUM eq “90” Then LBTPTNUM = 4, If TPTNUM eq “120” Then LBTPTNUM = 5	Perm	Timing

STEP 14

CDISC ADaM

Organizations have started implementation of the standards from Clinical Data Interchange Standards Consortium (CDISC). One of the key sets of standards is Analysis Data Model (ADaM), which is used for submitting analysis datasets, to the US Food and Drug Administration (FDA).

When implementing ADaM standards, much effort is focused on how to document and maintain analysis dataset specifications, as well as how to generate accurate analysis datasets.

There is a separate specification file for each analysis dataset, with the analysis file name as the specification file name.

The advantages of this approach for analysis data documentation are:

- Having a central location for all analysis dataset specifications
- Can be used as basis for independent validation for analysis datasets
- Easy to maintain changes or updates to the specifications

The metadata information will be programmatically turned into ATTRIB statements and KEEP statements, which are invoked by the analysis dataset program. This keeps the analysis attributes of dataset variables in sync with the specifications

Structure of Analysis dataset Specifications

- Variable Name
- Variable Label
- Type (Char or Num)
- Data Type (text, float, or integer)
- Length of variable

- Format
- Code list Name
- Origin of Existing Variable
- ADaM Define Specification (Logic for derivation)
- Role
- Core
- Comment

After finalizing the statistical analysis plan (SAP), analysis specifications are drafted. One way to ensure all the analysis variables are included in appropriate analysis datasets is to annotate mock-shells with the names of analysis dataset and variables that will be used for summary Tables, Figures, and Listings. By annotation, a SAS programmer / Analyst will determine the variable attributes.

In referencing annotated case report forms (CRFs), protocols, and SAPs, the source data name and source variable names that will be used to derive the analysis variables can be identified.

Once the type of data structure, type of variables, source data, and derivations are determined, specifications can be developed.

With implementation of ADaM standards, we use the following analysis data specifications. The specifications for analysis datasets are stored in a spreadsheet.

ADSL Specification:

Name	*Label*	*Type*	*Length*	*Origin*	*Derivation*
STUDYID	Study Identifier	Char	15	DM.STUDYID	
USUBJID	Unique Subject Identifier	Char	25	DM.USUBJID	
SUBJID	Subject Identifier for the Study	Char	25	DM.SUBJID	
SITEID	Study Site Identifier	Char	25	DM.SITEID	
COUNTRY	Country	Char	3	DM.COUNTRY	
INVNAM	Investigator Name	Char	200	DM.INVNAM	
SAER	Sex/Age/Ethnicity/Race	Char	200		
CONSDTC	Date of Informed Consent	Char	19		DS.DSSTDTC where (DS.DSCAT = 'PROTOCOL MILESTONE' and DS. DSDECOD = 'INFORMED CONSENT OBTAINED')
CONSDT	Date of Informed Consent (Num)	Num	8		Date part of CONSDTC converted to SAS numeric date
CONSDY	Day of Informed Consent	Num	8		CONSDY=CONSDT-TRTSDT+(CONSDT>=TRTSDT)

ENRLFL	Enrolled Analysis Set Flag	Char	1		If DS.Usubjid ne ‘’ Then enrlfl=”Y”; Elseenrlfl=’N’;
SAFFL	Safety Analysis Set Flag	Char	1		If subject had at least one non-missing EX.EXSTDTC Then SAFFL=”Y” ElseSAFFL=”N”
SAFEXC	Reason Excluded From Safety Pop.	Char	25		If SAFFL=”N” Then do the following: SAFEXC=”Not Dosed” If subject had all values of EX.EXSTDTC missing and no values of EXDOSE > 0 SAFEXC=”No Safety Assessments” If subject had all missing values of AE.AESTDTC, LB.LBORRES, EG. EGORRES, VS.VSORRES
EFFFL	Efficacy Analysis Set Flag	Char	1		If subject had at least one non-missing EX.EXSTDTC and the patient has value of XR.XTSTRESC where XR.XRTESTCD = ‘DISRESP’ Then EFFFL = ‘Y’. If SAFFL = ‘N’ or Value of XR.XRSTRESC is missing and (DS.DSSCAT=””END OF TREATMENT”” and DSREASN ne . or If the patient died) Then EFFFL = ‘N’

EFFEXC	Reason Excluded From Efficacy Pop.	Char	25		If EFFFL="N" Then do the following: EFFEXC="Not in Safety Population" If SAFFL="N" EFFEXC="Efficacy data not present"
TRT01P	Planned Study Treatment	Char	40		
TRT01PN	Planned Study Treatment Number	Num	8		
TRT01A	Actual Study Treatment	Char	40		trt01a= Put (trt01a, Trtfmt.);
TRT01AN	Actual Study Treatment Number	Num	8		
MTD	Maximum Tolerated Dose Level	Num	8		Coded for MTD against the treatment identified by the sponsor
AGE	Age	Num	8	DM.AGE	
AGEU	Age Units	Char	6	DM.AGEU	
AAGE	Age in Yrs at Informed Consent (Derived)	Num	8		AAGE=INT((ADSL.CONSDT - ADSL.BRTHDT) / 365.25));

AAGEGRN	Age Group 1 (Num)	Num	1		If . < AAGE<=65 Then AAGEGR1N =0; Else If AAGE>65 Then AAGEGR1N=1
SEX	Sex	Char	1	DM.SEX	
SEXN	Sex Code	Num	8		If SEX=»F» Then SEXN=0; Else If SEX="M" Then SEXN=1; Else null;
RACE	Race	Char	40	DM.RACE	
RACEN	Race (Num)	Num	8		If RACE='AMERICAN INDIAN OR ALASKA NATIVE' Then RACEN=1 ; If RACE='BLACK OR AFRICAN AMERICAN' Then RACEN=2 ; If RACE='WHITE' Then RACEN=3 ; If RACE='ASIAN' Then RACEN=4 ; If RACE='NATIVE HAWAIIAN OR OTHER PACIFIC ISLANDER' Then RACEN=5 ; If RACE='OTHER' Then RACEN=99 ;
RACEOTH	Race, Other	Char	200		If SC.SCTESTCD='RACEOTH' Then RACEOTH=SC.SCORRES

ETHNIC	Ethnicity	Char	40	DM.ETHNIC	
ETHNICN	Ethnicity (Num)	Num	8		If ETHNIC='HISPANIC OR LATINO' Then ETHNICN=1 If ETHNIC='NOT HISPANIC OR LATINO' Then ETHNICN=2 Else missing
TRTSDTC	Date/Time of First Exposure to Trt	Char	19		The earliest non-missing EX.EXSTDTC
TRTSDTM	Date/Time of First Exposure to Trt (Num)	Num	8		Convert TRTSDTC to SAS numeric date. Note: If time is missing, impute to "00:00:00". If only seconds are missing, Then impute seconds to "00".
TRTSDT	Date of First Exposure to Trt (Num)	Num	8		Datepart of TRTSDTM
TRTEDTC	Date/Time of Last Exposure to Trt	Char	19		The latest non-missing EX.EXENDTC
TRTEDTM	Date/Time of Last Exposure to Trt (Num)	Num	8		Convert TRTEDTC to SAS numeric date. Note: If time is missing, impute to "23:59:59". If only seconds are missing, Then impute seconds to "59".

TRTEDT	Date of Last Exposure to Trt (Num)	Num	8		Datepart of TRTEDTM
BRTHDTC	Date of Birth	Char	19	DM.BRTHDTC	
BRTHDT	Date of Birth (Num)	Num	8		Datepart of BRTHDTC converted to SAS numeric date
HEIGHTBL	Height at Baseline (cm)	Num	8		HEIGHTBL=VS.VSSTRESN and VSTESTCD="HEIGHT". This is the latest non-missing value of VS.VSSTRESN such that VSDTC <= TRTSDT. Order by usubjid, vsdtc, vsseq and take last non-missing value.
WEIGHTBL	Weight at Baseline (kg)	Num	8		WEIGHTBL=VS.VSSTRESN and VSTESTCD="WEIGHT". This is the latest non-missing value of VS.VSSTRESN such that VSDTC <= TRTSDT.
BMIBL	BMI at Baseline	Num	8		BMI is calculated as weightbl (kg)/heightbl^2(m^2) or weightbl (kg)/heightbl^2((cm/100)^2) depending on the unit of weight

SYSBPBL	Systolic Blood Pressure at Baseline	Num	8		SYSBPBL=VS.VSSTRESN and VSTESTCD=”SYSBP”. This is the latest non-missing value of VS.VSSTRESN such that VSDTC <= TRTSDT. Order by Usubjid, Vsdtc, Vsseq and take last non-missing value.
DIABPBL	Diastolic Blood Pressure at Baseline	Num	8		DIABPBL=VS.VSSTRESN and VSTESTCD=”DIABP”. This is the latest non-missing value of VS.VSSTRESN such that VSDTC <= TRTSDT.
TEMPBL	Temperate at Baseline	Num	8		TEMPBL=VS.VSSTRESN and VSTESTCD=”TEMP”. This is the latest non-missing value of VS.VSSTRESN such that VSDTC <= TRTSDT. Order by Usubjid, Vsdtc, Vsseq and take last non-missing value.
HRBL	Heart Rate at Baseline	Num	8		HRBL=VS.VSSTRESN and VSTESTCD=”HR”. This is the latest non-missing value of VS.VSSTRESN such that VSDTC <= TRTSDT.

COMPL	Did Patient Complete Study?	Char	1		If the subject has a record in DS such that DSSCAT=”END OF TREATMENT” and DSTERM=”COMPLETED” and DSDECOD=”COMPLETED” and the subject has a record in XQ that XQCAT=”END OF TREATMENT” and XQQRRES=’Y’ and XQTESTCD=’COMPLTYN’ Then COMPL=”Y”; Else COMPL=’N’;
DISCYN	Was Subject Discontinued From Study?	Char	1		If the subject has a record in DS such that DSSCAT=”END OF TREATMENT” and DS.DSDECOD in (“Adverse Event” , “Death (Accidental or Unknown Reason)”, “Requirement for therapy excluded by the protocol”, “Subject Non-Compliance”, “Subject Request”, “Investigator Request”, “Lost to Follow-up”, “Resistant Disease or Disease Progression”, “Other (Specify)”) Then DISCYN=”Y”; Else DISCYN=”N”;

DSREAS	Discontinued from Study Reason	Char	200		w "Subject Non-Compliance", "Subject Request", "Investigator Request", "Lost to Follow-up", "Disease Progression", "Other") If dsdecod= 'Advese Event' and suppds. aedltyn='Y' Then DSREAS= 'Advese Event - DLT'; Else If dsdecod ='Advese Event' and suppds. aedltyn='N' Then
					DSREAS='Advese Event - Other'; Else If dsdecod='Requirement for therapy excluded by the protocol' the dsreas= 'Excluded Therapy'; Else If dsdecod= 'Resistant Disease or Disease Progression' Then dsreas='Disease Progression'; Else If dsdecod='Other (specify)' Then dsreas= 'Other'; Else dsreas=dsdecod;

DSREASN	Discontinued from Study Reason (Num)	Num	8		If dsreas='Adverse Event – DLT' Then dsreasn=1; Else If dsreas='Adverse Event – Other ' Then dsreasn=2; Else If dsreas= 'Death (Accidental or Unknown Reason)' Then dsreasn=3; Else If dsreas='Excluded Therapy' Then dsreasn=4; Else If dsreas= 'Subject Non-Compliance' Then dsreasn =5; Else If dsreas='Subject Request' Then dsreasn=6; Else If dsreas= 'Investigator Request' Then dsreasn=7; Else If
					dsreas= 'Lost to Follow-up' Then dsreasn=8; Else If dsreas='Disease Progression ' Then dsreasn=9; Else If dsreas='Lost to Follow-up' Then dsreasn=99;
AEDLT	AE Related Dose Limiting Toxicity	Char	1		Defined only for DS.DSSCAT = "END OF TREATMENT" and DS.DSDECOD = 'ADVERSE EVENT' SUPPDS.QVAL where DS.DSSEQ and SUPPDS. QNAM='AEDLTYN'
DISDTC	Date of Discontinuation	Char	19		DISDTC=DS.DSSTDTC where DS.DSSCAT="END OF TREATMENT" and DSREASN ne .;

DISDT	Date of Discontinuation (Num)	Num	8		Convert DISDTC to SAS numeric date
DISDY	Day of Discontinuation	Num	8		DISDY=DISDT-TRTSTDT+1
LCDT	Last Contact Date	Num	8		Consider the following options. If patient died, Then get the Date of Death from DS. If the patient is alive Then 1) where DS.DSSCAT="SURVIVAL STATUS" and dsdecod = 'ALIVE'; the latest DS.DSSTDTC 2) latest date from SV. Take the maximum date from these dates If the patient is alive.
STDYDURD	Duration of Exposure (Days)	Num	8		STDYDURD=TRTEDT-TRTSDT+(TRTEDT>=TRTSDT)
DTHDTC	Date of Death	Char	19		DTHDTC=DS.DSSTDTC where DS.DSSCAT="Death";
DTHDT	Date of Death (Num)	Num	8		Convert DISDTC to SAS numeric date
DTHDAY	Day of Death	Num	8		DTHDAY=DTHDT-TRTSTDT+1
DTHREAS	Cause of Death	Char	200		DTHREAS=DS.DSDECOD C where DS.DSSCAT="Death";

DTHREASO	Primary Cause of Death, Specify	Char	200		DTHREASO=DS.DETERM where DS.DSSCAT=”Death” and index(DS. DSDECOD)=”Other”;
ARMCD	Planned Arm Code	Char	8	DM.ARMCD	
ARM	Description of Planned Arm	Char	40	DM.ARM	
INCFAIL	Failed Inclusion Criteria	Char	200		INCFAIL = (all inclusion criteria numbers where IE.IEORRES=”N” concatenated and separated by commas)
EXCFAIL	Failed Exclusion Criteria	Char	200		EXCFAIL=(all exclusion criteria numbers where IE.IEORRES=”Y” concatenated and separated by commas)

ADAE Specifications:

Name	Label	Type	Length	Origin	Derivation
STUDYID	Study Identifier	Char	15	ADSL.STUDYID	
USUBJID	Unique Subject Identifier	Char	25	ADSL.USUBJID	
SUBJID	Subject Identifier for the Study	Char	25	ADSL.SUBJID	
SITEID	Study Site Identifier	Char	25	ADSL.SITEID	
SAER	Sex/Age/Ethnicity/ Race	Char	200	ADSL.SAER	
AAGE	Age in Years at Informed Consent (Derived)	Num	8	ADSL.AAGE	
RACE	Race	Char	40	ADSL.RACE	
SEX	Sex	Char	1	ADSL.SEX	
ENRLFL	Enrolled Flag	Char	1	ADSL.ENRLFL	
SAFFL	Safety Analysis Set Flag	Char	1	ADSL.SAFFL	
EFFFL	Efficacy Analysis Set Flag	Char	1	ADSL.EFFFL	

TRT01P	Planned Study Treatment	Char	40	ADSL.TRT01P	
TRT01PN	Planned Study Treatment Number	Num	8	ADSL.TRT01PN	
TRT01A	Actual Study Treatment	Char	40	ADSL.TRT01A	
TRT01AN	Actual Study Treatment Number	Num	8	ADSL.TRT01AN	
TRTSDT	Date of First Exposure to Trt (Num)	Num	8	ADSL.TRTSDT	
TRTSDTM	Date/Time of First Exposure to Treatment (Num)	Num	8	ADSL.TRTSDTM	
TRTEDT	Date of Last Exposure to Trt (Num)	Num	8	ADSL.TRTEDT	
TRTEDTM	Date/Time of Last Exposure to Treatment (Num)	Num	8	ADSL.TRTEDTM	
AESEQ	Sequence Number	Num	8	AE.AESEQ	
AESTDTC	Start Date/Time of Adverse Event	Char	19	AE.AESTDTC	

AESTDT	Start Date of Adverse Event (Num)	Num	8		Datepart of AE.AESTDTC converted to SAS numeric date
AESTDY	Relative Day of AE Start Date	Num	8		If AESTDT GE TRTSTDT Then AESTDY=AESTDT - TRTSTDT +1 Otherwise AESTDY = AESTDT - TRTSTDT
AEENDTC	End Date/Time of Adverse Event	Char	19	AE.AEENDTC	
AEENDT	End Date of Adverse Event (Num)	Num	8		Datepart of AE.AEENDTC converted to SAS numeric date
AENDY	Relative Day of AE End Date	Num	8		AENDY=AEENDT - TRTSTDT + (AEENDT GE TRTSTDT)
AEDUR	Duration of AE	Num	8		AEENDT - AESTDT + 1
AETERM	Reported Term for the Adverse Event	Char	200	AE.AETERM	
AEDECOD	Dictionary-Derived Term	Char	200	AE.AEDECOD	
AEPTCD	Dictionary-Derived Term (Code)	Num	8		Numeric value of SUPPAE.QVAL where SUPPAE. QNAM="AEPTCD" (matching IDVARVAL on AESEQ)

AEBODSYS	Body System or Organ Class	Char	200	AE.AEBODSYS	
AELLT	Lowest Level Term	Char	200		SUPPAE.QVAL where SUPPAE.QNAM=”AELLT” (matching IDVARVAL on AESEQ)
AEHLT	High Level Term	Char	200		SUPPAE.QVAL where SUPPAE.QNAM=”AEHLT” (matching IDVARVAL on AESEQ)
AEHLGT	High Level Group Term	Char	200		SUPPAE.QVAL where SUPPAE. QNAM=”AEHLGT” (matching IDVARVAL on AESEQ)
AESER	Serious Event	Char	1	AE.AESER	
AEACN	Action Taken with Study Treatment	Char	40	AE.AEACN	
AEACNOTH	Other Action Term	Char	40	AE.AEACNOTH	
AEREL	Relationship to Study Drug	Char	40	AE.AEREL	
AEOUT	Outcome of Adverse Event	Char	60	AE.AEOUT	AEOUT = AE.AEOUT If AE.AEOUT ne ‘’ AEOUT = SUPPQUAL.QVAL If SUPPAE.QNAM = ‘AEOUTOTH’ and SUPPQUAL.AESEQ=AE. AESEQ and AE.USUBJID = SUPPQUAL.USUBJID

AESCONG	Congenital Anomaly or Birth Defect	Char	1	AE.AESCONG	
AESDISAB	Persist or Sign If Disability/Incapacity	Char	1	AE.AESDISAB	
AESDTH	Results in Death	Char	1	AE.AESDTH	
AESHOSP	Requires or Prolongs Hospitalization	Char	1	AE.AESHOSP	
AESLIFE	Is Life Threatening	Char	1	AE.AESLIFE	
AESMIE	Other Medically Imp. Serious Event	Char	1	AE.AESMIE	
AETOXGR	Standard Toxicity Grade	Char	40	AE.AETOXGR	
AEDTOX	Dose Limiting Toxicity	Char	1	SUPPAE.DOSETOXC	If AE.USUBJID= SUPPQUAL.USUBJID and AE.AESEQ=SUPPAE.AESEQ and SUPPAE.QNAM = 'DOSETOXC'

ADCM Specifications:

Name	*Label*	*Type*	*Length*	*Origin*	*Derivation*
STUDYID	Study Identifier	Char	15	ADSL.STUDYID	
USUBJID	Unique Subject Identifier	Char	25	ADSL.USUBJID	
SUBJID	Subject Identifier for the Study	Char	25	ADSL.SUBJID	
SITEID	Study Site Identifier	Char	25	ADSL.SITEID	
SAER	Sex/Age/Ethnicity/Race	Char	200	ADSL.SAER	
AAGE	Age in Years at Informed Consent (Derived)	Num	8	ADSL.AAGE	
RACE	Race	Char	40	ADSL.RACE	
SEX	Sex	Char	1	ADSL.SEX	
EFFFL	Efficacy Analysis Set Flag	Char	1	ADSL.EFFFL	
SAFFL	Safety Analysis Set Flag	Char	1	ADSL.SAFFL	
EFFFL	Efficacy Population Flag	Char	1	ADSL.EFFFL	
TRT01P	Planned Study Treatment	Char	40	ADSL.TRT01P	
TRT01PN	Planned Study Treatment Number	Num	8	ADSL.TRT01PN	
TRT01A	Actual Study Treatment	Char	40	ADSL.TRT01A	
TRT01AN	Actual Study Treatment Number	Num	8	ADSL.TRT01AN	

TRTSDT	Date of First Exposure to Trt (Num)	Num	8	ADSL.TRTSDT	
TRTSDTM	Date/Time of First Exposure to Treatment (Num)	Num	8	ADSL.TRTSDTM	
TRTEDT	Date of Last Exposure to Trt (Num)	Num	8	ADSL.TRTEDT	
TRTEDTM	Date/Time of Last Exposure to Treatment (Num)	Num	8	ADSL.TRTEDTM	
CMSEQ	Sequence Number	Num	8	CM.CMSEQ	
CMCAT	Category for Medication	Char	40		CM.CMCAT where CM.CMCAT in (“CONCOMITANT MEDICATIONS”, “PRIOR RADIIOTHERAPY”, “PRIOR SYSTEMIC THERAPY”, “ANCILLARY PROCEDURES”)
CMTRT	Reported Name of Drug, Med, or Therapy	Char	200	CM.CMTRT	
CMDECOD	Standardized Medication Name	Char	200	CM.CMDECOD	
PT	Preferred Term	Char	200		PT = scan(CM.CMDECOD,1,byte(183));
ATC1	Dictionary Term ATC1	Char	200		SUPPCM.QVAL where SUPPCM. QNAM=ATCTXT1

ATC1CD	Dictionary Code ATC1	Char	15		SUPPCM.QVAL where SUPPCM. QNAM=ATCCD1
ATC2	Dictionary Term ATC2	Char	200		SUPPCM.QVAL where SUPPCM. QNAM=ATCTXT2
ATC2CD	Dictionary Code ATC2	Char	15		SUPPCM.QVAL where SUPPCM. QNAM=ATCCD2
ATC3	Dictionary Term ATC3	Char	200		SUPPCM.QVAL where SUPPCM. QNAM=ATCTXT3
ATC3CD	Dictionary Code -ATC3	Char	15		SUPPCM.QVAL where SUPPCM. QNAM=ATCCD3
ATC4	Dictionary Term ATC4	Char	200		SUPPCM.QVAL where SUPPCM. QNAM=ATCTXT4
ATC4CD	Dictionary Code -ATC4	Char	15		SUPPCM.QVAL where SUPPCM. QNAM=ATCCD4
CMDOSTXT	Dose Description	Char	40	CM.CMDOSTXT	
CMDOSU	Dose Units	Char	20	CM.CMDOSU	
CMROUTE	Route of Administration	Char	40	CM.CMROUTE	
CMRTEOT	Route of Administration - Other	Char	40	CM.CMROUTE	SUPPCM.QVAL where SUPPCM. QNAM="ROUTEOTH" (matching IDVARVAL on CMSEQ)
CMLOC	Anatomical Location	Char	200		SUPPCM.QVAL where SUPPCM. QNAM="RADSITE" (matching IDVARVAL on CMSEQ)
CMGRPID	Regimen Number	Char	200	CM.CMGRPID	

CMINDC	Indication	Char	200	CM.CMINDC	
CMONGO	Ongoing	Char	1		Defined only for cmcat='CONCOMITANT MEDICATIONS' or cmcat="PRIOR SYSTEMIC THERAPY" If CM.CMENRTPT='ONGOING' Then CMONGO='Y'; ElseCMONGO='N';
CMRESP	Best Response	Char	200		SUPPCM.QVAL where SUPPCM.QNAM="BESTRSP1" or SUPPCM.QNAM="BESTRSP2" (matching IDVARVAL on CMSEQ)
RELAPSDT	Date of Relapse	Char	19		Defined only for cmcat = "PRIOR SYSTEMIC THERAPY"
					SUPPCM.QVAL where SUPPCM.QNAM="RELAPSDT" (matching IDVARVAL on CMSEQ)
CMREAS	Reason for Medication	Char	25		SUPPCM.QVAL where SUPPCM.QNAM="REASONMD" or SUPPCM.QNAM="REASONAP" (matching IDVARVAL on CMSEQ)

PRIORFL	Analyzed Prior Record Flag	Char	1		Defined only for cmcat = 'CONCOMITANT MEDICATIONS'. If CMSTDTC gt . and datepart (CMSTDTC) < datepart (ADSL.TRTSDTM) Then PRIORFL='Y'; ElsePRIORFL='N'. For partial dates, If month and year or only year value is present Then If month and year or year is less than or equal to month and year of ADLS.TRTSDTM Then PRIORFL = 'Y' Else PRIORFL = 'N'. If a subject is not in the Safety Population (SAFFL="N"), Then all CM records for that subject will have PRIORFL as null;
CONCOMFL	Analyzed Conmed Record Flag	Char	1		Defined only for cmcat= 'CONCOMITANT MEDICATIONS'. If CMONGO = 'Y' or (CMSTDTC ne . and datepart(CMSTDTC) >= datepart(ADSL.TRTSDTM) and da tepart(CMSTDTC)<=datepart(ADSL. TRTEDTM)) + 30 or (CMSTDTC ne . and Datepart (CMSTDTC) < Datepart (ADSL. TRTSDTM) and (datepart (CMENDTC) >= Datepart (ADSL>TRTSDTM) or datepart (CMENDTC) = .)) Then CONCOMFL='Y'; Else CONCOMFL='N';

					For partial dates, If month and year or only year value is present Then: If month and year or year is less than or equal to month and year of ADSL.
					If a subject is not in the Safety Population (SAFFL="N"), Then all CM records for that subject will have CONCOMFL as null;
PRCONFL	Analyzed Prior and Conmed Flag	Char	1		If PRIORFL = 'Y' and CONCOMFL = 'Y' Then PRCONFL = 'Y'
CMSTDTC	Start Date/Time of Medication	Char	19	CM.CMSTDTC	
CMSTDY	Start Day of Medication	Num	8	CM.CMSTDY	
CMENDTC	End Date/Time of Medication	Char	19	CM.CMENDTC	
CMENDY	End Day of Medication	Num	8	CM.CMENDY	

ADLB Specifications:

Variable Name	*Label*	*Type*	*Length*	*Origin*	*Derivation*
STUDYID	Study Identifier	Char	15	ADSL.STUDYID	
USUBJID	Unique Subject Identifier	Char	25	ADSL.USUBJID	
SUBJID	Subject Identifier for the Study	Char	25	ADSL.SUBJID	
SITEID	Study Site Identifier	Char	25	ADSL.SITEID	
SAER	Sex/Age/Ethnicity/Race	Char	200	ADSL.SAER	
AAGE	Age in Years at Informed Consent (Derived)	Num	8	ADSL.AAGE	
RACE	Race	Char	40	ADSL.RACE	
SEX	Sex	Char	1	ADSL.SEX	
ENRLFL	Enrolled Flag	Char	1	ADSL.ENRLFL	
SAFFL	Safety Analysis Set Flag	Char	1	ADSL.SAFFL	
EFFFL	Efficacy Analysis Set Flag	Char	1	ADSL.EFFFL	
TRT01P	Planned Study Treatment	Char	40	ADSL.TRT01P	
TRT01PN	Planned Study Treatment Number	Num	8	ADSL.TRT01PN	
TRT01A	Actual Study Treatment	Char	40	ADSL.TRT01A	
TRT01AN	Actual Study Treatment Number	Num	8	ADSL.TRT01AN	

TRTSDT	Date of First Exposure to Trt (Num)	Num	8	ADSL.TRTSDT	
TRTSDTM	Date/Time of First Exposure to Treatment (Num)	Num	8	ADSL.TRTSDTM	
TRTEDT	Date of Last Exposure to Trt (Num)	Num	8	ADSL.TRTEDT	
TRTEDTM	Date/Time of Last Exposure to Treatment (Num)	Num	8	ADSL.TRTEDTM	
LBSEQ	Sequence Number	Num	8	LB.LBSEQ	
LBREFID	Specimen ID	Char	40	LB.LBREFID	
PARCAT1	Parameter Category	Char	40	LB.LBCAT	PARCAT=LB.LBCAT
PARAMCD	Parameter Code	Char	8	LB.LBTESTCD	PARAMCD=LB.LBTESTCD
PARAM	Parameter Description	Char	60	LB.LBTEST	PARAM=LB.LBTEST|| " (||LB. LBSTRESU||")"
AVAL	Analysis Value	Num	8		Sort by USUBJID, LBTEST, VISIT, LBDTC, LBSEQ. If last.LBTDTC Then AVAL=LB. LBSTRESN
AVALC	Analysis Value (C)	Char	200		Sort by USUBJID, LBTEST, VISIT, LBDTC, LBSEQ. If last.LBTDTC Then AVALC=LB. LBSTRESC

DTYPE	Derivation Type	Char	8		For the Minimum Post-baseline Value and Maximum Post-baseline Value records, When AVISIT=Minimum Post-baseline Value and AVISITN=1000 Then DTYPE=MIN When AVISIT= Maximum Post-
					baseline Value and AVISITN=1001 Then DTYPE=MAX.
LBNRIND	Reference Range Indicator	Char	40	LB.LBNRIND	
BASE	Baseline Value	Num	8		For each USUBJID, LBTEST: BASE is the latest non-missing value of AVAL where (LBDY<=1) and (LBDTC<TRTSDTC) Note: Check date imputations for missing times. If missing time for trtsdtc or lbdtc Then use lbdy<=1 only.
ABLFL	Baseline Record Flag	Char	1		For each USUBJID, LBTEST: ABLFL="Y" for the record corresponding to the latest non-missing value of AVAL where LBDY<=1
CHG	Change from Baseline	Num	8		CHG=AVAL-BASE

BTOXFL	Baseline Toxicity Flag	Char	1		For each USUBJID, LBTOX: BTOXFL=”Y” for the record corresponding to the latest value of LBTOXGR where (LBDY<=1) and (LBDTC<TRTSDTC). Check date imputations for missing times. If missing time for trtstdtc or lbdtc Then use lbdy<=1 only.
BTOXGR	Baseline Toxicity Grade	Char	8		BTOXGR=LBTOXGR where BTOXFL=”Y”
CELLPCNT	Cell Percentage	Char	20		Select SUPPLB.QVAL where SUPPLB.QNAM=”CELLPRCNT” (matching on IDVARVAL and LBSEQ) For CYTOMETRY evaluations only
LBNAM	Vendor Name	Char	60	LB.LBNAM	
LBNAMSTD	Vendor Name Abbreviated	Char	60		LBNAMSTD=put (lbnam,$labnmf.); If aval ne . and LBNAMSTD is null Then LBNAMSTD=’MISSING’;
LBORRES	Character Result/Finding in Original Units	Char	200	LB.LBORRES	
LBORRESU	Original Units	Char	20	LB.LBORRESU	
LBORNRLO	Reference Range Lower Limit-Orig Units	Char	200	LB.LBORNRLO	
LBORNRHI	Reference Range Upper Limit-Orig Units	Char	20	LB.LBORNRHI	

LBSTRESN	Numeric Result/Finding in Standard Units	Num	8	LB.LBSTRESN	
LBSTRESC	Character Result/Finding in Std Format	Char	200	LB.LBSTRESC	If lb.lbstat = 'NOT DONE' Then for LBCAT = 'CYTOMETRY' place vlaue of LBREASND into LBSTRESC. Otherwise place value of LBSTAT into LBSTRESC
LBSTRESU	Standard Units	Char	20	LB.LBSTRESU	
LBCRESN2	Character Result/Finding in Converted Format	Char	200		If conversion value in the conversion factor excel file exists Then value is the calculated value of lbstren * conversion factor; otherwise it is the value of lbstresn
LBCRESU2	Converted Units	Char	20		If conversion value in the conversion factor excel file exists Then value is the converted standard unit presented in the file; otherwise it is the value of lbstresu
LBTOXGR	Standard Toxicity Grade	Char	8	LB.LBTOXGR	
LBSTNRLO	Reference Range Lower Limit-Std Units	Num	8	LB.LBSTNRLO	
LBSTNRHI	Reference Range Upper Limit-Std Units	Num	8	LB.LBSTNRHI	
LBDTC	Date/Time of Specimen Collection	Char	19	LB.LBDTC	

LBDT	Date of Specimen Collection	Num	8		Convert the Datepart of LBDTC into a SAS numeric date
LBDY	Study Day of Specimen Collection	Num	8	LB.LBDY	
VISIT	Visit Name	Char	40	LB.VISIT	
VISITNUM	Visit Number	Num	8	LB.VISITNUM	
AVISIT	Analysis Visit	Char	40	LB.VISIT	LB.VISIT Please add additional records for Minimum Post-baseline Value (AVISIT=Minimum Post-baseline Value) and Maximum Post-baseline Value(AVISIT=Maximum Post-baseline Value) for the parameters belonging to LBCAT HEMATOLOGY,CHEMISTRY and URINALYSIS where we have non-missing AVAL. Please take the most recent value for ADT, ADY, ADT, ADTM, LBSEQ amongst equal values for the Minimum Post-baseline Value and Maximum Post-baseline Value records.
AVISITN	Analysis Visit Numeric	Num	8	LB.VISITNUM	AVISITN=LB.VISITNUM. When AVISIT=Minimum Post-baseline Value Then AVISITN=1000 When AVISIT= Maximum Post-baseline Value Then AVISITN=1001
CRFORD	Order of tests according to CRF	Num	8		Number assigned to the tests according to their appearance in the CRF

Data Definition Tables (Define.pdf)

One of the elements of a successful FDA electronic submission is the data definition table (DDT). Three types of data definition tables are needed for a submission: 1) a list of all datasets and what type of information each contains (eg: Adverse Events, Demographics, etc.); 2) for each dataset in the database, a list of all variables, with variable type, variable format, and, if the variable is derived, algorithm; and 3) an alphabetical list of all the variables in the database, along with the dataset in which each resides.

The FDA requires a number of items relating to the transfer of data in support of a submission to the agency: SAS transport format files of each dataset, with a size of 25MB or less (uncompressed); case report tabulations; annotated CRFs (case report forms); data definition tables, etc. Many of us have had the experience of supplying these items to the FDA. One of the most cumbersome items is the data definition table, defined in Item 11.

DATA DEFINITION TABLES – DEFINED

Within Item 11, point 3 details what is expected in the documentation of datasets. The two PDF files required by the FDA and described in point 3 are define.pdf and blankcrf.pdf. Blankcrf.pdf contains the annotated CRFs, and define.pdf , the data definition tables. We will be discussing define.pdf. The data definition tables define all datasets in the database. Three types of data definition tables are requested:

- For all datasets, dataset name, description of the dataset, and location within the electronic submission of the transport file
- For each dataset, a table of all the variables, variable label, variable type, variable code, and variable comments
- An alphabetic list of all variables in the study datasets and the dataset in which each can be found.

Creating XPORT Transport files

Creating XPORT Transport file is the technique to transfer data files, catalogs, and/or applications between sites or operating environments. A transfer involves moving SAS entities between host environments. The entity could be a data set, a collection of data sets, a format catalog, or an application catalog.

For SAS data sets and catalogs, using transport files simplifies transfers between different operating systems or hardware platforms by providing a work-around for binary incompatibilities that exist because different computers store numbers differently. SAS transport file is a collection of one or more SAS data sets or catalog entries stored in transport format and stacked sequentially into a single file officially called a SAS transport library.

The most common situations that require transfers are:

- changing host environments, same location
- sharing work with other locations
- moving between companies or research groups
- upgrading to a later version of SAS software
- sharing with people stuck using an older release

Standard Transfer Process

The standard process for transfers is straightforward. The steps are as follows.

- Export: create transport file with source documentation
- QC: test export
- Move: transmit, or send physical media, with documentation
- Import: create SAS data set(s) from transport file
- QC: check new data sets using source documentation

Creating a Xport library: Xport Library is the place where XPORT files will be created

Libname Xptlib Xport 'E:\xport\ae.xpt';

Converting a SAS dataset to a Xport transport format by Proc Copy

Proc Copy in=YLP Out=Xptlib Memtype = data;

Select Events;

Run;

Converting .xpt file Back to SAS dataset*/

Proc Copy in=Xptlib Out=work;

Run;

Creating xpt files by Datastep

```
Data Xptlib.Xae;
Set YLP.Events;
Run;
```

Creating SAS datasets from xpt files by data step

```
Data Event;
Set Xptlib.Xae;
Run;
```

Proc Print to

Default Destinations for SAS Log and Procedure Output is the LOG window the OUTPUT window respectively. The Printto procedure allows you to specify destinations for SAS log and output files, instead of using the system defaults.

The syntax is as follows:

```
Filename Logfile 'D: \project\outputs\demo.log';
Filename Lisfile 'D: \project\outputs\demo.lst';
Proc Printto log=logfile print=lisfile new;
Run;
```

Here, the ***log file*** is rerouted to the Fileref called ***logfile*** and printed ***output*** is rerouted to the Fileref called ***lisfile***. Be aware that filename statements are highly system-dependent; the above example works for SAS operating under Windows but may not work for other operating systems.

The ***NEW*** parameter causes Proc Printto to start a new file; otherwise the procedure appends the new information to the bottom of the existing file.

PROC PRINTTO Statement

Tip: To reset the destination for the SAS log and procedure output to the default, use the PROC PRINTTO statement without options.

Tip: To route the SAS log and procedure output to the same file, specify the same file with both the LOG= and PRINT= options

**** SAS procedures go here;***

Proc Printto;

Run;

Proc Printto acts much like a switch. First, you turn it on, and then you have to turn it off again. In the above example, the first Proc Printto reroutes output to the two Filerefs, and the second Proc Printto closes the two output files and redirects output back to the default destinations. The two output files are then available for DATA step processing.

Give me six hours to chop down a tree and I will spend the first four sharpening the axe.

Abraham Lincoln

STEP 15

CREATING ANALYSIS DATASETS

The Analysis Data Sets (Value Added Datasets, Derived Datasets) used in the creation of Tables, Listings, and supporting Figures (TLFs) are key components to the accuracy, reliability and maintainability of a study. The variables and data sets must be carefully thought out while creating and are often subject to change at a later time as the clinical trial progresses and analysis goals become clearer.

Careful documentation of the derivation of the Analysis Variables, Analysis Dataset should be maintained and a consistent method to facilitate change control is essential for high-quality analyses.

While creating ADS, it is always better to prepare a Specifications document (Specs) which contains all the required Analysis Datasets to be prepared as well as Variables each Analysis dataset should contain.

Typically the Specs Document carries the following Information:

- Name of the ADS to be created
- Label of the ADS
- Input Datasets (Raw Datasets) required creating specific ADS
- Name, Label, Type, Length, Format of the Analysis Variables
- Source of the Analysis Variables (Raw Dataset Name, Derived, Assigned)

The key parameters for the specification of any derived variable

- Created Variable Name
- SAS Label
- Purpose
- Input SAS File
- Output SAS File

- Variables Needed
- Formats
- Length
- Type (Numeric or Character)
- Algorithm
- Quality Check
- Change Log (Modification history)

There are several benefits for such specifications:

Writing specifications is a proactive approach to design, plan and arriving at an efficient end result.

It makes one think through the problem to be solved more fully and analytically. Analysis database specifications force the writer to fully understand what data they are working with as raw material and what they are trying to express in the newly created variables and data sets used when programming the TLFs.

Variables and data sets which are well thought out and specified have a greater chance of working correctly than those which are hastily put into service. When there is a single source of algorithm/Procedure, which is well conceived and documented in the specification, future maintenance efforts are far more efficient.

Examples of some variables created while creating ADS

- Age --- Duration calculations
- ITTFL, SAFFL, COMPFL -- study populations
- RFSTDTC, AESTDTC -- Creating Time and Date variables (Imputing)
- DSREASN -- LOCF
- AVISIT, AVISITN --visit windowing
- LBSEQ, AESEQ -- Creating Sequence_Id
- PARAM, PARAMCD -- CONCATENTING/TRANSFORMING
- AVALC -- Conversions of Units
- ANRIND -- ASSIGNING FLAGS

We may need to use some of the following concepts while creating ADS

- Study Population / Analysis Population (SAF, ITT, PP)
- Study day calculations
- Transposing Datasets
- Duration calculations
- Visit windowing
- Creating Time and Date variables (Imputing)
- Baseline Definition ,Change From Baseline(CFB)
- Creating Flag Variables
- Creating Sequence Id
- TEAE Flagging
- Unit Conversions
- TIME TO EVENT calculations
- LOCF,BOCF
- Abnormal Indicator Flag (CS,NCS)

Study Populations / Analysis Populations:

- Efficacy analyses will be based on the intent-to-treat (ITT) analysis set. This population is defined as all patients randomized to study treatment.
- Safety analyses will be based on the Safety Population, defined as all enrolled patients receiving at least one dose of any study drug.
- The Per Protocol Set is defined as those patients in the ITT set who are compliant with the study protocol.
- The precise reasons for excluding patients from the Per Protocol Set will be clearly defined and documented before breaking the blind.

Study day Variable:

Time is a critical measure for clinical trial analysis Time is captured in clinical trial databases in a “study day” variable. Study day can be defined as the number of days from therapeutic intervention to any given time point or event.

By defining study day, you create a common metric for measuring time across a population of patients in a clinical trial. There can be a study day calculation for any time point of interest such as adverse event start, Study termination, and clinical endpoint event date etc.

The study day calculation is performed with one of the two following approaches.

- Study day calculations without day zero
- Study day calculations with day zero

Study day calculations without day zero:

If event of interest is less than initial intervention date

```
Data _null_;
Event_date='25Nov2011'D;
Iniintvdt='01Dec2011'D;
Studyday=Event_date - Iniintvdt;
Put Event_date= Iniintvdt= Studyday=;
Run;
```

If event of interest is greater than or equal to initial intervention date

```
Data _null_;
Event_date='05dec2011'd;
Iniintvdt='01dec2011'd;
Studyday=Event_date-iniintvdt+1;
Put Event_date= Iniintvdt= studyday=;
Run;
```

USE OF THE "STUDY DAY" VARIABLES

The permissible Study Day variables (--DY, --STDY, and --ENDY) describe the relative day of the observation starting with the reference date as Day 1.

They are determined by comparing the date portion of the respective date/time variables (--DTC, --STDTC, and --ENDTC) to the date portion of the Subject.

Reference Start Date (RFSTDTC from the Demographics domain)

The Subject Reference Start Date (RFSTDTC) is designated as Study Day 1. The Study Day value is incremented by 1 for each date following RFSTDTC. Dates prior to RFSTDTC are decremented by 1, with the date preceding RFSTDTC designated as Study Day -1 (there is no Study Day 0). This algorithm for determining Study Day is consistent with how people typically describe sequential days relative to a fixed reference point, but creates problems if used for mathematical calculations because it does not allow for a Day 0. As such, Study Day is not suited for use in subsequent numerical computations, such as calculating duration. The raw date values should be used rather than Study Day in those calculations.

You will find that you need to create --DY and or --STDY /--ENDY variables in almost all the SDTM domains. Because the Process of the derivation is same, it makes sense to create a macro code and use it across all the domains.

```
Data DM;
Input Subjid Rfstdtc $10.;
Datalines;
101 2013-12-25
102 2013-12-20
104 2014-01-02
;
Run;

Data Event;
Input Subjid Aestdtc $10.;
Datalines;
101 2014-01-25
102 2013-12-15
104 2014-01-28
;
Run;
```

```
Proc sort data=dm out=dm (keep=Subjid Rfstdtc);
By Subjid;
Run;

Proc Sort Data=Event;
By Subjid;
Run;

Data Test;
Merge Event (in=a) dm;
By Subjid;
If a;
Refdt_n = Input (Substr (Rfstdtc, 1, 10), yymmdd10.);
Eventdt_n = Input (Substr (Aestdtc, 1, 10), yymmdd10.);
If NMISS (Refdt_n, Eventdt_n) = 0 then
Aedy = Eventdt_n - Refdt_n +( Eventdt_n >= Refdt_n);
Run;
```

TASK: In a study, duration of taking a medication is 5 days and 5 mg of capsule need to be taken thrice a day. Subjects will be given placebo in pre-baseline visits. Subjects will be considered under efficacy evaluable population if the post baselines have more than 80% of the compliance with the study drug.

Please list down the subjects who will be included in the efficacy analysis and explain how, based on the data represented below

```
Data Test;
Input Subject Stdy doses_perday @@;
Datalines;
1001 -2 3 1001 -1 3 1001 1 2 1001 2 3 1001 3 1 1001 4 3 1001 5 1
1002 -2 1 1002 -1 1 1002 1 2 1002 2 3 1002 3 3 1002 4 3 1002 5 3
1003 -2 3 1003 -1 3 1003 1 0 1003 2 3 1003 3 3 1003 4 1 1003 5 3
;
Run;
```

Change from Baseline:

- Change from Baseline analysis is frequently used to evaluate the effect of medical intervention by comparing the measures of change from baseline in some clinical characteristic between treatment groups.
- Creating Changes from Baseline is common task in clinical data analysis since Change from Baseline helps clinical researchers to estimate the treatment effect.
- The baseline value is typically a measure of a clinical characteristic before the medical intervention, while the post baseline value is the measure at a defined time point or period after the intervention.

```
Data Vitals;
Input Patid Trt Visit height weight Visdate mmddyy10. @@;
Datalines;
101 1 1 173.45 70.2 01-02-2013 101 1 1.1 173.01 70.5 09-02-2013
101 1 1.2 173.49 71.4 09-04-2013 101 1 2 . . 09-06-2013
101 1 3 174.17 70.9 09-08-2013 101 1 4 173.60 65.1 09-10-2013
101 1 5 174.10 63.5 09-12-2013 201 2 1 182.45 88.7 09-02-2013
201 2 2 182.49 88.1 07-04-2013 201 2 3 183.12 80.4 06-06-2013
201 2 4 182.60 76.1 09-08-2013 201 2 5 182.15 74.2 10-10-2013
401 1 1 125.45 70.1 09-06-2013 401 1 2 125.49 68.5 07-08-2013
401 1 3 125.00 66.1 09-10-2013
;
Run;

Proc Means Data=Vitals (where = (1 <= visit <=2)) Noprint;
By patid;
Var weight;
Output out=BL(drop=_TYPE_ _FREQ_) mean=BLweight;
Run;
```

```
Proc means data=Vitals (where = (3 <= visit <=5)) Noprint;
By patid;
Var weight;
output out=WDT(drop=_TYPE_ _FREQ_) mean=Trtweight;
Run;

Data CFB;
Merge BL WDT;
By Patid;
Mean_Chg = Blweight - Trtweight;
Pct_Chg= (Blweight - Trtweight)/Blweight*100;
Run;
```

Visit Windowing:

Generally all clinical trials have to deal with 'unscheduled' or 'off cycle' visits and aligning them with the planned visits in order to make use of the data collected. Now our task is to align the data collected with the visit in which it was intended to occur.

For this we are going to use the approach of visit windows, given that a detailed visit schedule is provided with either the Protocol or Statistical Analysis Plan.

This detailed plan usually provides the study days throughout the study on which subjects should be at the investigators site for some type of assessment. Frequently this type of assessment occurs when subject dosing happens once at the beginning of the study or regularly for the duration of the study.

Once you have reviewed the Protocol and Statistical Analysis Plan and determined that the right approach is to use the visit window, the next step is to evaluate the data. Since visit windows are usually based on study days, the first step is to calculate the study days based on the specification in the SAP.

Once you have calculated the study days you would then perform a frequency evaluation on those days. Be aware that each type of data, such as laboratory or vital signs, may have different study day frequencies that will need to be evaluated.

As an example, let's evaluate the laboratory data:

→ Based on the SAP, the study days are based on number of days after a subject is randomized on the study, with the day of randomization being day 1.

→ Based on the protocol, the subject is supposed to show up every two weeks for 2 months. After you have calculated the study days, creating a frequency table on the study days for the WBC yields the results in Table. This gives you the basic data to identify the visit windows to be used for the study.

Based on our Protocol, you would expect the visits to happen on days 1, 12, 26, 40, and 54 or 2 days prior or later to the actual site visit.

However, in reviewing the data, you can tell that we have laboratory visits on day 10, 34 and 60. If you were to look at the data, you might also find that the recorded visits don't actually match to the visit schedule.

For the purposes of this example, we are just going to look at the visit frequencies, but be aware there may be other issues to consider. Once again, it is good to review this data with the study team to make sure you have taken into consideration all the potential permutations.

Based on the algorithm, we should probably schedule visit 1, or the baseline visit, to occur just on day 1. From there, visit two would occur from day 10 to 14, visit three on day 26 to 28, visit 4 on visit 34 to 42, and visit 5 on day 54 to 60. Notice that we are not including the days outside of the visit windows.

```
Data Labs;
Input Subjid Stdy Lbtest $10. lbrn @@;
Datalines;
101 -3 Hematocrit 41 101 1 Hematocrit 46 101 11 Hematocrit 48
101 13 Hematocrit 51 101 27 Hematocrit 45 101 29 Hematocrit 38
101 37 Hematocrit 33 101 56 Hematocrit 40 101 58 Hematocrit 47
;
Run;
```

```
Data LB_win;
Set Labs;
If -14 <= Stdy <= -7 then Visid=-2;
Else If -7 <= Stdy <= -1 then Visid=-1;
Else If Stdy = 1 then Visid = 1;
Else if 10 <= Stdy <= 14 then Visid=2;
Else if 26 <= Stdy <= 28 then Visid=3;
Else if 34 <= Stdy <= 38 then Visid=4;
Else if 54 <= Stdy <= 60 then Visid=5;
Else If Visid = . Then put "War" "ning: Visit window error" Stdy=;
Run;
```

Basic Lab Pre-Processing

1. Exclude lab records with status 'NOT DONE' before Processing, and bring them back at the end. It will save a lot of program running time and avoid some unexpected programming errors
2. Flag the records with missing Lab dates and report them to Data Management team for resolution
3. Identify records with duplicates and report them to Data Management team for resolution. These 'irregular' records should be cleaned before data base lock (DBL). They will cause unexpected programming errors.

Laboratory data yields some of the largest and most unwieldy data sets SAS programmers encounter in a project. Lab data usually is collected both on data collection forms (case report forms), and in an electronic format, such as a spreadsheet or text file straight from the lab. Extensive data manipulation is almost always required in order to get the data into a format that is useful for analysis, and to combine the other collected data with the data from labs correctly.

Harmonize names of panels and analyte

Lab data usually appears as a set of panels, and within each panel is a set of individual tests called analyte. Examples of panel names are Hematology, Chemistry, and Urinalysis. Examples of analyte names are Glucose, Potassium, and Red Blood Cell Count. There is not a regulatory standard for naming these panels or analyte, so if data comes in from more than one laboratory, one step the SAS programmer must complete is to "harmonize" the names of the panels and analyte so that the data sets can be appropriately mapped together. Generally, there are only a few panel names to deal with, and the project analyst may specify how panel names are to appear in titles in mock output, so harmonizing panel names is fairly straightforward. Individual analyte are another matter. One laboratory may abbreviate the lab analyte in the above example as "GLU", "K", "RBC". Another may concatenate the lab name with the units in parentheses such as "Glucose (mmol/L)", "Potassium (mmol/L)", RBC (10^12/L)". If a SAS programmer is faced with these different methods of naming analyte, he or she should create a new analyte name variable that is consistent for all labs.

Create numeric values from character values

Often one data set includes both a numeric and a character version of lab result values. In some cases these values are the same, such as a numeric 5 and a character '5'. But in other cases a numeric equivalent of the character value is not so obvious.

Some examples include character values such as: 'NA', 'N/A', 'ND', '<2.0', 'Below Limit of Quantization' (or 'BLQ'), 'Neg', 'Trace', and '+'. Usually for such values the numeric variable for this same record will have a missing value. Obviously numeric calculations that might be necessary to convert the original values to standard values cannot be performed on these character values as they are. Some analyte such as certain urine tests are not measured numerically so no conversion is expected (results are presented in frequency tables, not summary statistics). A clinician may have to make the final call as to whether or not the associated numeric value should always be treated as missing. For example, sometimes the decision is made to strip off any "<" or ">" and assign the remaining number as the numeric result. Or "BLQ" may be the same as "<0.7" for a particular lab machine, and this value may be analyzed as 0.7.

Multiple Measurements within a Visit Date

There are cases of the repeated measurements of the same test being done at the same date but the collection time is not in the database. The best solution is to use the average of the same date measurements. This will not bias to the result and will be consistent. The average value can be used for summary of the change from baseline.

The baseline value will be calculated from the last two measurements if there are multiple scans done on the same date, the average value will be used as a single input to the baseline calculation.

Dealing with Partial Dates:

A common occurrence with many Clinical Trials data is the collection of partial dates, when the full date is unknown. Partial dates make summarizing the data successfully and accurately more difficult and may impact the validity of the trial if not handled correctly.

The FDA states "Missing values represent a potential source of bias in a clinical trial. Hence every effort should be undertaken to fulfill the requirements of the protocol concerning the collection and management of data. In reality, however, there will almost always be some missing data. A trial may be regarded as valid, nonetheless, provided the methods of dealing with missing values are sensible, particularly if those methods are predefined in the protocol". This guidance goes on to state "no universally applicable methods of handling missing values can be recommended.

Dates are an integral part of the data collected within clinical trials. Visits, investigational product doses, adverse events and medical history are just a few common data types where dates are often used. However, alongside the obvious advantages of date collection is the common occurrence of missing and partial dates, where the complete date is not known. As stated above by the FDA Guidance, these situations need to be handled in a robust manner and documented accordingly.

A partial start date with a missing start day, e.g. - -JUN2013, will often be set to the first of the month, 01JUN2013. If the month is missing e.g. 15- - -2013, the month will often be set to January for that year, 15JAN2013.

The reverse is often true for a partial end date, with the missing day set to the end of the month and the missing month set to December. Consideration needs to be taken with partial end dates with missing days, to ensure that months having differing number of days are taken into account.

Special care also needs to be applied with February because of the extra day included in leap years. If there is only a year and both the day and month are missing, then both are imputed, giving 1st January for a start date or 31st December for a stop date.

Time to Event Analysis

Time-to-event analysis in clinical trials is concerned with comparing the distributions of time to some event for various treatment regimens.

The two nonparametric tests used to compare distributions are

1. Log-rank test
2. ***Cox proportional hazards model.*** (The Cox proportional hazards model is more useful when you need to adjust your model for covariates)

During oncology studies, a typical measure of efficacy is the amount of time elapsed until a particular response is achieved for the first time (time to response) and how long that response is maintained (duration of response)

- For subjects that do not meet the response criteria before the end of the study, a censoring flag and time must also be calculated

Time-to-event parameters are an important component in determining the safety and efficacy of a drug during a clinical trial. Since the derivation of these parameters typically utilizes multiple data points across several domains and time points, calculations can be complex and difficult to program. An additional complication is the inclusion of a censoring variable that is used for subjects that do not meet the criteria of the event.

One event of interest in a large percentage of studies is the response of the subject to the study medication.

Response is usually collected on a case report form (CRF) at the end of each treatment cycle and is separated into several different levels (e.g. partial response, complete response, SD.)

It may also depend on other parameters like tumor size and laboratory assessments. Each study will have slightly different criteria for when a positive response is achieved. Some important parameters to calculate is time to response (TTR) which is defined as the time elapsed between some starting points at the beginning of the study usually date of first dosing, and the day on which the positive response was first achieved.

Another important parameter is the duration of response (DOR) which is the time between the date of the first positive response and relapse.

Additional parameters of interest may be the best level of response achieved and the time to each individual level of response.

Normally, not all subjects in a study achieve a positive response, but most analyses (e.g. Kaplan–Meier) require that the days spent in the study by the non-responding subjects are counted.

This is accomplished by censoring subjects on the last day they were in the study (or some other end point) and giving them a time-to-event duration equal to the number of days from first dosing to the censoring date.

A binary censoring variable is then determined with one value for those that met the response criteria and the opposite value for those that are censored.

Note that the values for this variable will typically be 0 and 1 (a value of 1 will be given to those with the event and a value of 0 to those who were censored).

Thus, the end result of deriving a time-to-event parameter should be a data set containing the time-to-event duration variable and the censor variable for each subject.

Duration of Response

- Another important parameter in determining the efficacy of a study drug is how long a positive response is maintained once it is achieved.
- It is defined as the number of days between the date when response was achieved and the date when the subject either relapses or ends the study.

Determining value for VISFWDID in Adverse Events:

There should be no unscheduled visits in the EVENTS ADS. A separate record should be created for each visit at which an event is present as recorded on the Events CRF. A visit identifier is related to the start date of an event on the CRF, so that visit identifier is the starting VISFWDID. If the event end date is the same as the visit date, then select the later of:

- The visit identifier of the visit date
- The last visit identifier recorded on the CRF (if the subject left the office and had the event, it should be recorded as occurring on the next visit).

If AE start date is between Visit N and N+1 dates and AE end date is between Visit M and M+ 1 date, then we create records with VISFWDID from N+1 to M+1 by AEID.

If the event starts after the final visit (VISIT.VISFWDID) then map the event to the last visit.

Imputation for incomplete Start Dates for the derivation of VISFWDID:

- If year, month, and day are missing then use the minimum of the subjects first visit date (VISIT.VISDT) or the consent date.
- If either only month or month and day are missing then use January 1.
- If only day is missing then use 1 for the first day of the month.

Imputation for incomplete End Dates for the derivation of VISFWDID:

- If year, month, and day are missing then use the subjects last visit date (VISIT.VISDT).
- If either only month or month and day are missing then use December 31.
- If only day is missing then use the last day of the month.

Proc Transpose (Transposing Datasets)

Clinical trial data, there are two types of datasets

- Normalized dataset (Vertical)
- Non-Normalized dataset (Horizontal)

The shape in which we obtain the dataset is defined by the underlying CRF design.

Most commonly we get Normalized datasets which are perfectly suitable for analyzing a variable.

When we want to perform analysis on observation we need to reshape or ***re-organize*** the dataset, for this we use ***Proc Transpose***.

Transposes are limited to two types, and a combination of these two. It would be a lot easier if these observations were next to each other, describes an 'up' transpose. "Up" transposes can be thought of changing rows of a dataset to columns, or changing a vertical data structure to a horizontal data structure.

It would be a lot easier if these variables were observations one underneath each other", describes a "down" transpose. "Down" transposes can be thought of as changing columns to rows, or changing a horizontal data structure to a vertical data structure.

After having determined whether your transpose is an "Up" or "Down", you need to ask yourself four questions.

- ✦ What should stay the same?
- ✦ What goes up?
- ✦ What goes down?
- ✦ What goes into the middle?

Answering these questions will lead us to build our PROC TRANSPOSE syntax as per our requirement.

```
Data Tran;

Input usubjid visit Val$ leuc lymph @@;

Datalines;

1 1 VAL1 48.60 88.63 1 1 VAL2 35.28 56.60 1 1 VAL3 38.66 28.91

1 2 VAL1 39.29 53.01 1 2 VAL2 97.34 56.64 1 2 VAL3 30.71 74.91

1 3 VAL1 68.08 29.79 1 3 VAL2 68.73 57.30 1 3 VAL3 95.54 61.51

2 1 VAL1 15.96 68.73 2 1 VAL2 81.96 55.49 2 1 VAL3 18.10 96.86

2 2 VAL1 27.80 93.18 2 2 VAL2 16.88 30.92 2 2 VAL3 69.98 51.48

2 3 VAL1 35.55 30.02 2 3 VAL2 40.81 84.36 2 3 VAL3 33.03 90.69

;

Run;
```

In Proc Transpose we use the following statements:

By Statement:

In your data set, there should be variables that you want to keep in your output data set. Variables that need to be kept in their original structure should be specified in the BY statement.

If you are doing an "Up" transpose, these variables need to identify unique values of your "Up" variable. These variables are USUBJID and VISIT. We can think of the rest of the transpose as rotating the data set around these variables.

```
Data Tranmod;
Set Tran;
Keep usubjid visit val;
Run;
PROC TRANSPOSE DATA=tranmod OUT=tranall;
RUN;
```

By default all the numeric variables would be transposed that means all the responses in the numeric variables will be converted to new variables.

If we want to keep some variables structure same like in the original dataset we use BY statement.

```
PROC TRANSPOSE DATA=tranmod OUT=tranby;
BY usubjid;
RUN;
```

ID statement:

We have already determined that there is an "Up" element to this transpose, and that ***Val*** is going up. But what does this mean? This means that the individual values of ***Val*** are to be turned into variables themselves. One variable for each unique value of ***Val*** will be created.

```
PROC TRANSPOSE DATA=Tran OUT=tranout;
BY Usubjid Visit;
ID Val;
Run;
```

VAR statement:

The VAR statement performs two distinct movements: Down, and Middle.

```
PROC TRANSPOSE DATA=tran OUT=tranvar;
BY Usubjid Visit;
ID Val;
VAR Leuc Lymph;
Run;
```

```
Data Lab;
Input Subjid Visit Lbtest $ Lbrn @@;
Datalines;
101 1 leukocyte 14.2 101 2 leukocyte 15.2 101 3 leukocyte 14.8 101 4 leukocyte 15.5
101 1 lymphocyte 6.7 101 2 lymphocyte 6.4 101 3 lymphocyte 5.4 101 4 lymphocyte 6.5
102 1 leukocyte 14.2 102 2 leukocyte 14.5 102 3 leukocyte 13.8 102 4 leukocyte 15.6
102 1 lymphocyte 6.2 102 2 lymphocyte 6.4 102 3 lymphocyte 5.4 102 4 lymphocyte 6.8
;
Run;
```

By executing the above step we created a normalized dataset which contains 4 variables and 16 obs

```
Proc sort Data=Lab Out=Labsrt;
By Subjid Lbtest;
Run;
```

```
Proc Transpose Data=Labsrt out=Labflt prefix=vis;
By subjid lbtest;
Id visit;
Run;
```

Flagging Concomitant Medications

Medication start and stop dates will be compared to the date of first dose of study medication to allow medications to be classified as either Prior, Prior and Concomitant, or Concomitant. Medications starting after the completion/withdrawal date will be listed but will not be classified or summarized.

Medications that start and stop prior to the date of first dose of study medication will be classified as Prior medications. If a medication starts before the date of first dose of study medication and stops on or after the date of first dose of study medication then the medication will be classified as Prior and Concomitant.

Medications will be classified as Concomitant if they have a start date on or after the date of first dose of study medication. If medication start and/or stop dates are missing or partial, the dates will be compared as far as possible with the date of first dose of study medication.

Medications will be assumed to be concomitant, unless there is clear evidence (through comparison of partial dates) to suggest that the medication started prior to the first dose of study medication.

```
Data infcon;
Input id icdt ddmmyy10.;
Datalines;
101 23-12-2011102 12-12-2011103 11-11-2011104 11-12-2012
;
Run;

Data drdose;
Input id drstdt ddmmyy10. +1 drendt ddmmyy10.;
Datalines;
101 20-12-2011 21-12-2011
102 15-12-2011 25-12-2011
103 07-11-2011 08-11-2011
104 08-12-2011 16-12-2011
;
Run;
```

Task: Project the drug as prior med, conmed, prior and conmed based on prior med -- before joining the trial, Conmed -- after joining the trial, prior and conmed -- started prior to joining the trial but continued even in trial.

TEAE Flag

The correct identification of treatment-emergent adverse events is pivotal to the safety and efficacy of a study. The precise definitions of treatment-emergent adverse events may vary between different studies. Typically, the intent is to identify adverse events that begin during treatment as treatment-emergent, a treatment-emergent adverse event can indicate that the study drug is causing a harmful effect.

Considerations of TEAE:

- ✦ Assign treatment emergent flag for AEs that started on or after first dose date.
- ✦ For events that started before first dose date but continue on study, see if the severity increased compared to baseline severity.

Creating Dose date info dataset

```
Data Strdt;
Set YLP.Sdytrt;
Keep Subjid Visid Sdydosedt;
Run;
```

Sort the resultant dataset by invid subjid sdydosedt

```
Proc Sort Data=Strdt out=Strdtt;
By  Subjid Sdydosedt;
Run;
```

Create a dataset which contains only one record with dosestdt per subject

```
Data Strdtm;
Set strdtt;
By invid subjid;
If first.subjid;
Run;
```

Creating the AE Dataset:

```
Data Ae;
Set YLP.Events;
Keep Subjid Pterm Aestdt Aesev;
Run;

Proc Sort Data=Ae out=Aereq;
By Patid Socterm Pterm Aesev;
Run;
```

Merge this dataset with Aereq

```
Data aefin;
Merge Aereq (in=a) strdtm (in=b);
By Patid;
If a;
Run;
```

Assign treatment emergent flag for AE's that started on or after first dose date

```
Data Aefinal;
Set aefin;
If aestdt ne . and sdydosedt ne . and aestdt ge sdydosedt then teaefl = 1;
else teaefl = 0;
Run

Data aefinal1;
Set aefinal;
Where teaefl=1;
Run;
```

For events that started before first dose date but continue on study, see if the severity increased compared to baseline severity

```
Data basesev;
Set aefinal;
If aestdt ne . and sdydosedt ne . and
aestdt lt sdydosedt and Visid <= 3 and Aesev ne .;
Run;
```

Sort the resultant dataset by Patid pterm aesev

```
Proc sort data=basesev out=basesev;
by Patid pterm aesev;
Run;

data bsevfin;
set basesev;
by Patid pterm aesev;
if last.pterm;
basesev=aesev;
keep patid  pterm basesev;
Run;
```

LOCF

Laboratory tests have to be performed at each visit as per the study design and lab result has to be collected on a particular day.

Analysis of lab data has to be performed for each scheduled visit in the study. Each scheduled visit is required to occur on a specific study day for each patient and there is no room provided for these visits. Despite of following GCP guidelines by sites, many patients missed to visit the site on the day they should have visited and so collection of data falls on unscheduled days. Even though such collected results are not for scheduled visits in the study, these results are important from analysis point of view and they should not be excluded from analysis. At the same time, data is missing for important time points in the study (Scheduled Visits) for analysis purpose. By carrying forward the non-missing results from the previous available visit of the patient, analysis can be performed.

We are interested in a lab result of each subject at each scheduled visit.

- Last Observation Carried Forward is a frequently used and a popular imputation (is the Process of replacing missing data with substituted values.) method used in the pharmaceutical industry.
- If a patient drops out of the study after second week, then the value is 'carried forward' until the end of the treatment, as a conservative estimate of how well the subject would have done if remained in the study.

In another application, a vital signs dataset contains an observation for each time a patient has a scheduled/ unscheduled visit with a doctor. If a patient missed an assigned visit, then the primary measure is missing.

We will be considering the weight, as measurement of interest. LOCF imputation would use non-missing weight from an early visit as the weight for the later missing visit.

Below is a SAS code that generates four distinct patients with 1 to 4 distinct visits and random measurements for weight. A couple of patients have missing weight information such as patient 1 at visits 2 and 3, patient 2 at visit 3, patient 3 at visit 2 and patient 4 at visits 1 and 3. We can use LOCF methods to retain the non-missing weight measurement from an early visit if the weight measurement for current visit is missing.

```
Data Test;
Input Patid Visit Weight @@;
Datalines;
1 1 122 1 2 . 1 3 . 1 4 123
2 1 156 2 3 . 3 1 112 3 2 .
4 1 . 4 2 123 4 3 .
;
Run;
```

Please note that patient 4 is missing weight information at visit 1. When applying LOCF methods we need to make sure, the correct information for the correct patient is being carried forward from the non-missing visits.

It uses a RETAIN statement to create a temporary variable called tempval. This variable will retain the value that needs to be imputed from one patient to another .

The only drawback of this Procedure is the assumption that the baseline value (visit 1) will always be non-missing.

```
data all;
do i=1 to 4;
do j=1 to 4;
Patid=i;
visit=j;
output;
end;
end;
drop i j;
Run;
```

The dataset includes four patients, each one being assigned a number of four scheduled visits for a total of sixteen observations.

```
Proc Sort Data=Test;
By Patid visit;
Run;

Proc Sort Data=all;
By Patid visit;
Run;
```

Below we will RETAIN tempval as 0.

```
Data Final (drop=tempval);
Retain tempval 0;
Merge Test (in=b) all (in=all);
By Patid visit ;
If all;
If weight eq . then weight=tempval;
Else tempval=weight;
Run;
```

```
Data final3;
Set Test;
By Patid visit;
array reset(*) lagx1-lagx3;
lagx1=lag(weight);
lagx2=lag2(weight);
lagx3=lag3(weight);
if first.Patid then count=1;
do i=count to dim(reset);
reset(i)=.;
end;
count+1;
if weight=. and lagx1 ne . then weight=lagx1;
else if weight=. and lagx1 eq . and lagx2 ne . then weight=lagx2;
else if weight=. and lagx1 eq . and lagx2 eq . then weight=lagx3;
Run;
```

FIRST STEP – sort data set sda by patient and by visit. This way, the appropriate weight measurements will be used for LAGN () function in the data step.

SECOND STEP - define the array 'reset' by declaring the number of missing variables per patient. As a general rule, we should have a total of n-1 array elements (where n equals total number of possible or scheduled visits). In our case, n is 4 as total possible visits. The reason behind this logic is that we need to carry forward for a maximum number of possible visits less one (the original observation we use as primary for our LOCF).

THIRD STEP – set to missing the array 'reset' – lagx1, lagx2, lagx3 each time first observation for a patient occurs.

This way, we prevent a weight measurement being carried forward from one patient to another.

FOURTH STEP - we need to consider all LAGN () for weight values we need to carry forward from one visit to another.

For example, if weight is missing for a particular visit and lagx1 is not missing, then we use lagx1 value to populate the current missing weight measurement. In another case, if the current weight and lagx1 are missing, then we use the earliest non-missing measurement available – either one lagx2, or lagx3.

It is a good idea to know there are multiple ways to obtain LOCF results because it encourages SAS programmers to become more creative while programming their code. Before starting LOCF, we need to ask ourselves what is the final dataset we want to obtain. Do we want to generate a common dataset with all the possible values for scheduled visits, or are we interested only in LOCF values for missing measurements in the dataset of interest to us? After we answer this question, we need to check the structure of our data and chose the most efficient method that produces accurate results. The most important thing to mention about LOCF is that we need to be familiar with our data.

If we are not cautious enough, we could impute incorrect information to different patients or time points and that could affect the integrity of the information to be analyzed.

Duration Calculation

Calculation of duration is common in clinical reporting. Often in clinical trials, the start dates and stop dates of adverse events or of medication usage are recorded. Clinical programmers are required to compute the number of distinct days in these time intervals for each subject. When a subject has multiple time intervals, gaps and overlaps in these time intervals can be a major challenge in duration calculation.

In clinical trials, a subject may have experienced multiple adverse events (AEs) with different degrees of severity or may have taken multiple medications of different dosages at various time intervals.

Subject 101 has experienced adverse events in four different time intervals. Some of these time intervals overlap each other. One is entirely embedded within another interval. Another, the last interval, is disjoint from other intervals. Because of overlaps and gaps among intervals, one cannot compute the number of distinct days by simply adding the total number of days in each interval. In this example, the actual number of distinct days with adverse events is 26, however, by adding number of days in each interval, the total number of days is 34! In other words, the duration has been inflated by 8 days

```
Data Ae_dur;
Input SUBJID STARTDATE date9. +1 STOPDATE date9.;
Datalines;
101 01JAN2013 09JAN2013
101 05JAN2013 20JAN2013
101 16JAN2013 18JAN2013
101 26JAN2013 31JAN2013
;
Run;
```

A vertical representation of Adverse Events data is commonly used in clinical trials. This normalized data representation enables clinical data managers to easily record adverse events records regardless of the number of adverse events per subject.

For some methods of duration calculation, it will be easier to have a dataset like AE_DURH below --- a horizontal representation of the AE_DUR data set, using repeated fields for start dates and stop dates. The major challenge of this data representation is to know the number of repeated fields needed before the actual data collection. Hence, this representation is seldom used in clinical data collection. Rather, a horizontal data representation is often achieved by manipulating the vertical data representation.

Transpose data from Vertical Representation to Horizontal Representation.

```
Proc Sort Data=AE_DUR;
By SUBJID STARTDATE;
Run;
Proc Transpose Data=AE_DUR out=STARTDT (drop=_name_) prefix=START;
By SUBJID;
Var Startdate;
Run;
```

```
Proc Transpose data=AE_DUR out=STOPDT (drop=_name_) prefix=STOP;
By SUBJID;
Var STOPDATE;
Run;

Data AE_DURH;
Merge STARTDT STOPDT;
By SUBJID;
Run;
```

Simply Counting: Generate an observation for each date within any interval

```
data AE_DURR;
set AE_DUR; *--- Use Vertical Data Representation. ---*;
do XDATE=STARTDATE to STOPDATE;
output;
end;
Run;
```

Count only the distinct dates within any intervals.

```
Proc sql noprint;
Create table AE_D as
Select SUBJID, count (distinct XDATE) as DURATION label='Duration|(Days)'
From AE_DURR
Group by SUBJID
Order by SUBJID
;
Quit;
Proc Print Data=AE_D label split='|';
Var SUBJID DURATION;
Run;
```

TABLE Shells

Programmers, when programming Tables, Listings or Figures (TLFs) for a clinical trial, often begin with a diagram or shell of how the display should look. Programmers need to identify the elements that are needed to produce the TLF display.

While Creating a Table, Listing or Graph we need to check the following things:

- What is the main variable being analyzed and how?
- What is the population?
- What variables are displayed?
- Does the data come from one data set or many?
- What values are displaying? – Summary statistics, counts, confidence intervals, p-values?
- What procedures will we need to analyze the data?

After checking the above things we need to Review specific documents like Protocol, SAP and Specifications which gives us useful information for creating a Report.

CLINITRIAL CRO
Protocol WHY-EL-08

Table 1
Summary of Disposition
(Randomized Subjects)

	Placebo (N=xx)	1 mg (N=xx)	3 mg (N=xx)	6 mg (N=xx)	Total (N=xxx)
Total Number of Patients					
Safety	xx (xx.x%)	xx (xx.x%)	xx (xx.x%)	xx (xx.x%)	xx (xx.x%)
Intent-to-Treat	xx (xx.x%)	xx (xx.x%)	xx (xx.x%)	xx (xx.x%)	xx (xx.x%)
Modified Intent-to-Treat	xx (xx.x%)	xx (xx.x%)	xx (xx.x%)	xx (xx.x%)	xx (xx.x%)
Per Protocol	xx (xx.x%)	xx (xx.x%)	xx (xx.x%)	xx (xx.x%)	xx (xx.x%)
Number of Patients					
Completed	xx (xx.x%)	xx (xx.x%)	xx (xx.x%)	xx (xx.x%)	xx (xx.x%)
Early Terminated	xx (xx.x%)	xx (xx.x%)	xx (xx.x%)	xx (xx.x%)	xx (xx.x%)
Early Termination Reasons					
Adverse Event	xx (xx.x%)	xx (xx.x%)	xx (xx.x%)	xx (xx.x%)	xx (xx.x%)
Inclusion/Exclusion not met	xx (xx.x%)	xx (xx.x%)	xx (xx.x%)	xx (xx.x%)	xx (xx.x%)
Investigator Decision	xx (xx.x%)	xx (xx.x%)	xx (xx.x%)	xx (xx.x%)	xx (xx.x%)
Lack of Efficacy	xx (xx.x%)	xx (xx.x%)	xx (xx.x%)	xx (xx.x%)	xx (xx.x%)

Lost to Follow Up	xx (xx.x%)	xx (xx.x%)	xx (xx.x%)	xx (xx.x%)	xx (xx.x%)
Patient Died	xx (xx.x%)	xx (xx.x%)	xx (xx.x%)	xx (xx.x%)	xx (xx.x%)
Protocol Violation	xx (xx.x%)	xx (xx.x%)	xx (xx.x%)	xx (xx.x%)	xx (xx.x%)

CLINITRIAL CRO
Protocol WHY-EL-08

Table 2
Demographics and Baseline Characteristics
(ITT Population)

	Placebo (N=xx)	1 mg (N=xx)	3 mg (N=xx)	6 mg (N=xx)	Total (N=xxx)
Age (years) (1)					
Number of Patients	xx	xx	xx	xx	xx
Mean (SD)	xx.x (xx.xx)	xx.x (xx.xx)	xx.x (xx.xx)	xx.x (xx.xx)	xx.x (xx.xx)
Median	xx.x	xx.x	xx.x	xx.x	xx.x
Min, Max	xx.x, xx.x	xx.x, xx.x	xx.x, xx.x	xx.x, xx.x	xx.x, xx.x
Age Class (years)					
Number of Patients	xx	xx	xx	xx	xx
< 65	xx (xx.x%)	xx (xx.x%)	xx (xx.x%)	xx (xx.x%)	xx (xx.x%)
> 65	xx (xx.x%)	xx (xx.x%)	xx (xx.x%)	xx (xx.x%)	xx (xx.x%)
Gender					
Number of Patients	xx	xx	xx	xx	xx
Male	xx (xx.x%)	xx (xx.x%)	xx (xx.x%)	xx (xx.x%)	xx (xx.x%)
Female	xx (xx.x%)	xx (xx.x%)	xx (xx.x%)	xx (xx.x%)	xx (xx.x%)

Note: Percentages are based on the number of patients with data available in each treatment group.

CLINITRIAL CRO

Protocol WHY-EL-08

Page x of n

Table 6

Concomitant Medications

(ITT Population)

	Placebo	1 mg	3 mg	6 mg	Total
	(N=xx)	(N=xx)	(N=xx)	(N=xx)	(N=xxx)
Number of Patients With at	xx (xx.x%)	xx (xx.x%)	xx (xx.x%)	xx (xx.x%)	xx (xx.x%)
Least One Concomitant Medication					
Drug Class	xx (xx.x%)	xx (xx.x%)	xx (xx.x%)	xx (xx.x%)	xx(xx.x%)
Preferred Term #1	xx (xx.x%)	xx (xx.x%)	xx (xx.x%)	xx (xx.x%)	xx (xx.x%)
Preferred Term #2	xx (xx.x%)	xx (xx.x%)	xx (xx.x%)	xx (xx.x%)	xx (xx.x%)
Preferred Term #3	xx (xx.x%)	xx (xx.x%)	xx (xx.x%)	xx (xx.x%)	xx (xx.x%)
Drug Class	xx (xx.x%)	xx (xx.x%)	xx (xx.x%)	xx (xx.x%)	xx (xx.x%)
Preferred Term #1	xx (xx.x%)	xx (xx.x%)	xx (xx.x%)	xx (xx.x%)	xx (xx.x%)
Preferred Term #2	xx (xx.x%)	xx (xx.x%)	xx (xx.x%)	xx (xx.x%)	xx (xx.x%)
Preferred Term #3	xx (xx.x%)	xx (xx.x%)	xx (xx.x%)	xx (xx.x%)	xx (xx.x%)

CLINITRIAL CRO
Protocol WHY-EL-08

Page x of n

Table 16
Change from Baseline in HbA1c (%) – Efficacy Analysis (ANCOVA)
(mITT Population)

Timepoint	Placebo (N=xx)	1 mg (N=xx)	3 mg (N=xx)	6 mg (N=xx)
....				
Visit 15				
No of Patients	xx	xx	xx	xx
Mean (SD)	xx.x (xx.xx)	xx.x (xx.xx)	xx.x (xx.xx)	xx.x (xx.xx)
Median	xx.x	xx.x	xx.x	xx.x
Min, Max	xx.x, xx.x	xx.x, xx.x	xx.x, xx.x	xx.x, xx.x
Visit 15 CFB				
No of Patients	xx	xx	xx	xx
Mean (SD)	xx.x (xx.xx)	xx.x (xx.xx)	xx.x (xx.xx)	xx.x (xx.xx)
Median	xx.x	xx.x	xx.x	xx.x
Min, Max	xx.x, xx.x	xx.x, xx.x	xx.x, xx.x	xx.x, xx.x
LS Mean (SE)	xx.x (xx.xx)	xx.x (xx.xx)	xx.x (xx.xx)	xx.x (xx.xx)
LS Mean Diff. (90% CI)		xx.x (xx.x, xx.x)	xx.x (xx.x, xx.x)	xx.x (xx.x, xx.x)
p-value:		0.xxx	0.xxx	0.xxx

CLINITRIAL CRO

Protocol WHY-EL-08

Page x of n

Table 16

Change from Baseline in HbA1c (%) – Efficacy Analysis (ANCOVA)

(mITT Population)

	Placebo	1 mg	3 mg	6 mg
Timepoint	(N=xx)	(N=xx)	(N=xx)	(N=xx)
Endpoint (LOCF)				
No of Patients	xx	xx	xx	xx
Mean (SD)	xx.x (xx.xx)	xx.x (xx.xx)	xx.x (xx.xx)	xx.x (xx.xx)
Median	xx.x	xx.x	xx.x	xx.x
Min, Max	xx.x, xx.x	xx.x, xx.x	xx.x, xx.x	xx.x, xx.x
Endpoint (LOCF) CFB				
No of Patients	xx	xx	xx	xx
Mean (SD)	xx.x (xx.xx)	xx.x (xx.xx)	xx.x (xx.xx)	xx.x (xx.xx)
Median	xx.x	xx.x	xx.x	xx.x
Min, Max	xx.x, xx.x	xx.x, xx.x	xx.x, xx.x	xx.x, xx.x
LS Mean (SE)	xx.x (xx.xx)	xx.x (xx.xx)	xx.x (xx.xx)	xx.x (xx.xx)
LS Mean Diff. (90% CI)		xx.x (xx.x, xx.x)	xx.x (xx.x, xx.x)	xx.x (xx.x, xx.x)
p-value:		0.xxx	0.xxx	0.xxx

CLINITRIAL CRO

Page x of n

Protocol WHY-EL-08

Table 45

Treatment Emergent Adverse Events by System Organ Class and Preferred Term

(Safety Population)

System Organ Class	Placebo	1 mg	3 mg	6 mg	Total	
Preferred Term	(N=xxx)	(N=xx)	(N=xx)	(N=xx)	(N=xxx)	
Total Number of Treatment Emergent Adverse Events	xxx	xxx	xxx	xxx	xxx	
Number of Patients With at Least One Treatment Emergent Adverse Event	xx (xx.x%)	xx (xx.x%)	xx (xx.x%)	xx (xx.x%)	xx (xx.x%)	
System Organ Class 1	xx (xx.x%)	xx (xx.x%)	xx (xx.x%)	xx (xx.x%)	xx (xx.x%)	
Preferred Term 1	xx (xx.x%)	xx (xx.x%)	xx (xx.x%)	xx (xx.x%)	xx (xx.x%)	
Preferred Term 2	xx (xx.x%)	xx (xx.x%)	xx (xx.x%)	xx (xx.x%)	xx (xx.x%)	
System Organ Class 2	xx (xx.x%)	xx (xx.x%)	xx (xx.x%)	xx (xx.x%)	xx (xx.x%)	
Preferred Term 1	xx (xx.x%)	xx (xx.x%)	xx (xx.x%)	xx (xx.x%)	xx (xx.x%)	
Preferred Term 2	xx (xx.x%)	xx (xx.x%)	xx (xx.x%)	xx (xx.x%)	xx (xx.x%)	

CLINITRIAL CRO Page x of n

Protocol WHY-EL-08

Table 47

Possibly Study Drug Related Treatment Emergent Adverse Events by System Organ Class and Preferred Term (Safety Population)

System Organ Class	Placebo	1 mg	3 mg	6 mg	Total	
Preferred Term	(N=xxx)	(N=xx)	(N=xx)	(N=xx)	(N=xxx)	
Total Number of Treatment-Emergent Adverse Events	xx	xx	xx	xx	xx	
Related to Study Drug (1)	xx (xx.x%)	xx (xx.x%)	xx (xx.x%)	xx (xx.x%)	xx (xx.x%)	
Not Related to Study Drug (1)	xx (xx.x%)	xx (xx.x%)	xx (xx.x%)	xx (xx.x%)	xx (xx.x%)	
Number of Patients With at Least One						
Study Drug-Related Treatment-Emergent						
Adverse Event (2)	xx (xx.x%)	xx (xx.x%)	xx (xx.x%)	xx (xx.x%)	xx (xx.x%)	
System Organ Class 1	xx (xx.x%)	xx (xx.x%)	xx (xx.x%)	xx (xx.x%)	xx (xx.x%)	
Preferred Term 1	xx (xx.x%)	xx (xx.x%)	xx (xx.x%)	xx (xx.x%)	xx (xx.x%)	
Preferred Term 2	xx (xx.x%)	xx (xx.x%)	xx (xx.x%)	xx (xx.x%)	xx (xx.x%)	
Preferred Term 3	xx (xx.x%)	xx (xx.x%)	xx (xx.x%)	xx (xx.x%)	xx (xx.x%)	

CLINITRIAL CRO Page x of n

Protocol WHY-EL-08

Table 49

Treatment Emergent Adverse Events by Severity by System Organ Class and Preferred Term

(Safety Population)

System Organ Class		Placebo	1 mg	3 mg	6 mg	Total
Preferred Term	Intensity	(N=xxx)	(N=xx)	(N=xx)	(N=xx)	(N=xxx)
Number of Patients With at Least One Adverse Event		xx(xx.x%)	xx(xx.x%)	xx(xx.x%)	xx(xx.x%)	xx(xx.x%)
System Organ Class #1						
Preferred Term #1	Mild	xx(xx.x%)	xx(xx.x%)	xx(xx.x%)	xx(xx.x%)	xx(xx.x%)
	Moderate	xx(xx.x%)	xx(xx.x%)	xx(xx.x%)	xx(xx.x%)	xx(xx.x%)
	Severe	xx(xx.x%)	xx(xx.x%)	xx(xx.x%)	xx(xx.x%)	xx(xx.x%)
PREFERRED TERM #2	MILD	xx(xx.x%)	xx(xx.x%)	xx(xx.x%)	xx(xx.x%)	xx(xx.x%)
	MODERATE	xx(xx.x%)	xx(xx.x%)	xx(xx.x%)	xx(xx.x%)	xx(xx.x%)
	SEVERE	xx(xx.x%)	xx(xx.x%)	xx(xx.x%)	xx(xx.x%)	xx(xx.x%)

God has given you one face and
you make yourself another.

William Shakespeare

STEP 16

CREATING REPORTS

TABULATE Procedure

The presentation of data is an essential part of every clinical study, and SAS provides tools that enable the user to create a large variety of Reports. The Tabulate Procedure is a powerful and valuable Procedure that can be used in this Process. It can be used to create simple to highly customizable and flexible reports.

- ✦ Proc Tabulate is a Procedure that displays descriptive statistics in a tabular format.
- ✦ Proc Tabulate can produce up to three dimensional tables and allows within each dimension one or more variables are reported hierarchically.

Syntax of Proc Tabulate:

Proc Tabulate Options;

Var Variables;

Class Variables;

Tables Dimensions;

Run;

VAR Statement lists the analysis variables.

Analysis variables are always numeric and are used to compute statistics and arithmetic sums. Analysis variables tend to be continuous.

CLASS Statement lists the classification variables.

Classification variables contain values by which you want to summarize or group your data. Classification variables can be either character or numeric. Classification variables are best when they have discrete values.

TABLE statement defines the report table, what it contains, and what its structure will contain.

- ✦ It is the TABLE statement that requires a specific understanding in order to design and create a report.

Table Statement Syntax

Table Page definition, Row definition, Column Definition;

- ✦ Page definition --- Used only when the report is to span multiple pages
- ✦ Row definition --- Defines the rows of a report within a page
- ✦ Column definition --- Defines columns of a report
- ✦ The individual page, row, and column definitions are made up of building blocks and the building blocks are made up of items.
- ✦ The items can be Analysis Variables (Var statement), Classification variables (Class statement), formats, text, or options.

The building blocks themselves come in three forms:

- ✦ Singular the item appears by itself-→Table Race, Ageyr;
- ✦ Nested (two items are joined by an asterisk)→ Table Race*Sex, Ageyr;
- ✦ Concatenated two items are joined by a space →Table Race Sex, Ageyr;

Creating a Singular Table

Proc Tabulate Data=YLP.Dmads;

Var Ageyr;

Table Ageyr;

Run;

- ✦ The report has a single column, with the header AGE to identify the variable, and the header SUM to identify the Statistic.
- ✦ There is just a single table cell, which contains the value for the sum of AGE for all of the observations in the dataset Dmads.

Adding a Statistic:

If the variable in your table is an analysis variable, meaning that it is listed in a VAR statement, then the statistic you will get by default is the Sum.

- To specify the statistic for a Proc Tabulate table, you modify the TABLE statement. You list the statistic right after the variable name. To tell TABULATE that the statistic MEAN should be applied to the variable Ageyr, you use an asterisk to link the variable name to the statistic keyword.

```
Proc Tabulate Data=YLP. Dmads;
Var Ageyr;
Table Ageyr*MEAN;
Run;
```

- We can add similar code to our TABLE statement to get the number of observations, to add this statistic to the first table, all you do is combine the code for the mean (Age*MEAN) with the code you would used to get the number of observations (Age*N).
- The code for the two "Tables" is combined by using a space between the two statements. The space operator tells TABULATE that you want to add another column to your table.

```
Proc Tabulate Data= YLP.Dmads;
Var Ageyr;
Table Ageyr*N Ageyr*Mean;
Run;
```

- When SAS is creating a one dimensional table, additional variables, statistics, and categories are always added as new columns

Using Parentheses

To keep your table code easy to read, it is helpful to simplify it as much as possible. One thing you can do is use parentheses to avoid repeating elements in row or column definitions.

For example, instead of defining the table statement like this: TABLE Ageyr*N Ageyr*MEAN;

It can be defined like this: Table Ageyr*(N MEAN);

Adding a Classification Variable

- By specifying a variable to categorize your data, you can produce a concise table that shows values for various subgroups in your data. To break down Age by Sex, we will use Sex as a classification variable.
- By keeping the variable Sex in a CLASS statement, we are telling tabulate that the variable will be used to identify categories of the data.
- We do this by again using the asterisk operator. By adding another asterisk to the end of the TABLE statement, and following it with the variable name Sex. Tabulate knows that Sex will be used to categorize the mean values of Age.

```
Proc Tabulate Data= YLP.Dmads;
Class Sex;
Var Ageyr;
Table Ageyr*Mean*Sex;
Run;
```

Two-Dimensional Tables:

- To add another dimension to the table, you use a comma as an operator.
- All you do is put a comma between the row variable(s) and the column variable(s).
- If a Table statement has no commas, then it is assumed that the variables and statistics are to be created as columns.
- If a Table statement has two parts, separated by a comma, then tabulate builds a two dimensional table using the first part of the Table statement as the rows and the second part of the Table statement as the columns.

```
Proc Tabulate Data= YLP.Dmads;
Class Sex;
Var Ageyr;
Table Sex, Ageyr*Mean;
Run;
```

Adding Classification variables on both Dimensions

- With two dimensions, you can classify your statistics by two different variables at the same time. To do this, you put one classification variable in the row dimension and one classification in the column dimension.
- In the following code, we leave Sex as the row variable, and we leave age in the column dimension. The only change is to add Race to the column dimension using the asterisk operator. This tells Tabulate to break down each of the column elements into categories by Race.

```
Proc Tabulate Data= YLP.Dmads;
Class Sex Race;
Var Ageyr;
Table Sex, Ageyr*Race*Mean;
Run;
```

Adding another Classification Variable

- If we want to display additional subgroups of the data, we need to add Site as an additional row classification. The variable is added to the CLASS statement and to the row dimension of the TABLE statement.
- It is added using a space as the operator, so we will get rows for Sex followed by rows for Site.

```
Proc Tabulate Data= YLP.Dmads;
Class Sex Site Race;
Var Ageyr;
Table Site Sex, Ageyr*Race*Mean;
Run;
```

- We now have two two-dimensional mini-tables within a single table.
- First, we have a table of Age by Site and Race, and then we have a table showing Age by Sex and Race.
- This ability to stack multiple mini-tables within a single table can be a powerful tool for delivering large quantities of information in a user-friendly format.

Nesting the Classification variables

In the row definition if we put, the asterisk operator to show that we want to nest the two row variables. In other words, we want to see the breakdown of Age by Sex within each category of Site.

```
Proc Tabulate Data= YLP.Dmads;
Class Sex Site Race;
Var Ageyr;
Table Site*Sex, Ageyr*Race*Mean;
Run;
```

Adding Totals to the Rows and Columns

It is easy to generate Totals in Tabulate, simply use the ALL variable. You need not have to list it in the Class statement because it is a classification variable by definition.

- The following code produces a table with row totals. The statistic is changed to N so that you can see how the totals work.

```
Proc Tabulate Data= YLP.Dmads;
Class Sex Race;
Table Sex, (Race all)*n;
Run;
```

Three - Dimensional Tables

- A three-dimensional table looks like a two-dimensional table, except that it spans multiple pages.
- A one-dimensional table just has columns. A two-dimensional table has both columns and rows.

- A three-dimensional table is just a two-dimensional table that is repeated across multiple pages. You print a new page for each value of the page variable.

```
Proc Tabulate Data= YLP.Dmads;
Class Sex Site Race;
Var Ageyr;
Table Site, Trt (Sex All)*Ageyr*mean;
Run;
```

Making the Table Pretty

Notice how the totals column is titled 'All'. We can make this table more readable by changing that title to "Overall." To do this, we just attach the label to the keyword in the TABLE statement with an equal sign operator.

This operator is used to apply labels to variables and statistics.

```
Proc Tabulate Data= YLP.Dmads;
Class Sex Site Trt;
Var Ageyr;
Table Race, (Sex All='Over All')*Ageyr*Mean;
Run;
```

- Another thing that could be improved about this table is getting rid of the excessive column headings.
- We can get rid of the labels we attach a blank label.
- A blank label is two quotes with a single blank space in between. The blank label is attached to the variable using an equal sign.

```
Proc Tabulate Data= YLP. Dmads;
Class Sex Site Race;
Var Ageyr;
Table Race=' ', (Sex=' ' All='Over All')*Ageyr=' '*Mean=' ';
Run;
```

Notice that there is a big empty box above the rows and to the left of the column headings. This space (Row Title Space) can be used by specifying BOX= option, to hold a label describing our table.

Proc Tabulate Data= YLP.Dmads;

Class Sex Site Race;

Var Ageyr;

*Table Race=' ', (Sex=' ' All='Over All')*Ageyr=' '*Mean=' '/ Box='Average Age';*

Run;

Using Formats

You can use any of three primary ways to format the cells of a tabulate table.

- ✦ If a variable is already formatted or if you want to assign a format to a variable, the FORMAT statement can be used in TABULATE.
- ✦ You can also provide a default format for the numeric summarization cells on the PROC statement through the use of the FORMAT= option.
- ✦ You can use an asterisk to associate (nest) a format with a statistic.

Proc Format;

Value genfmt 1= 'Female' 2= 'Male';

Run;

Proc Tabulate Data=YLP.Dmads Format=8.3;

Class sex;

Var ageyr;

Table sex all, ageyr(n*f=3.0 mean stderr);*

Format sex genfmt.;

Run;

- ✦ Here a format has been created for use with the variable SEX. It is then assigned using the traditional FORMAT statement.
- ✦ The cells associated with the summary statistics (N MEAN MEDIAN) are given a default format (8.3) with the FORMAT= option to control the number of decimal places.
- ✦ Since N will be an integer, it should not have any decimal places, they are removed by associating the format 3.0 with that specific statistic.

Removing Repeated Text

The ROW= FLOAT option can be used to collapse the row header space when a statistic or constant text is nested within row definitions.

To remove the cells we use the ROW=FLOAT option. The FLOAT option removes columns that only contain blanks by dividing the RTS equally among non-blank columns.

Proc Tabulate Data=YLP.Dmads;

Class Site Sex;

Var Ageyr;

*Table Site*Ageyr=' '*Mean=' ', Sex /Row=float Box='Mean Weight';*

Run;

Replacing Missing Values

- A table created by TABULATE, may contain missing values. These may or may not accurately reflect what you want to have displayed.
- We can force the replacement of missing values using the MISSTEXT= option.
- MISSTEXT= Allows you to specify the character or text to print in empty cells instead of the '.' that SAS uses for missing numeric values.

Proc Tabulate YLP.Dmads;

Class Race Sex;

Var Ageyr;

*Table Race, Sex*Ageyr=' '*(n=' ' mean=' ') /Box='Mean Age' Misstext='No Value';*

Run;

Proc Report (REPORT Procedure)

The REPORT procedure combines features from the PRINT, MEANS, and TABULATE procedures with features of DATA step to provide a powerful report writing tool. It is frequently used in the pharmaceutical industry to create summary tables and listings.

In the Clinical Research and pharmaceutical industries, PROC REPORT is the method of choice to generate Tables and Listings. We can create Tables and Listings by Proc Tabulate, Proc Report or Data

Null. The method which you chose is based on the mock shell and client requirement/ specification.

- ✦ Proc Report is more user-friendly and the code easier to understand and consequently debug.
- ✦ Data _Null_ approach allows the users to create fully customize reports, but the code is little lengthy and complicated.

Let us have a look at the reporting output portion in our SAP, It states:

REPORTING OUTPUT:
✦ The REPORT Procedure will be used to produce all tables and listings whenever possible.
✦ Tables, listings will be produced as RTF files using ODS and Courier New font size 9.

By looking at this we can understand that we need to use Proc report to create Tables and Listings and should use ODS Facility to send the reports to RTF files.

Syntax of Proc Report

Proc Report Data= dataset name;

Column variable list and column specifications;

Define column / column usage options and attributes;

Compute column;

Compute block statements;

Endcomp;

Break statement / Options;

Rbreak statement / Options;

Run;

To create a report in an Interactive window:

Proc Report Data=YLP. Labs;

Run;

By submitting the above code we create a report in an interactive window (Proc Report window would be opened), in which we can reorganize the report as per our requirement and copy the source code, tweak it as per specification. But this approach is not discussed here since most of the programmers prefer coding approach (non interactive window).

To suppress the interactive window we use nowd, nowindows option

Proc Report Data= YLP. Labs Nowindows;

Run;

We can observe the following things in the report

- ✦ Simple Report doesn't have an OBS column
- ✦ The Variables are listed in their order in the Dataset
- ✦ The Column headers are the labels not the variable names
- ✦ The Column headers are adjusted to the column width

As a default, Proc Report uses the variable labels as column headings. This is different than Proc Print which uses variable names as column headings. If you want to create a report that uses variable names as column headings, the NOLABELS system option

OPTIONS NOLABEL;

Proc Report Data= YLP. Labs Nowindows;

Run;

Using the Column Statement

- ✦ The COLUMN statement is used not only to identify the variables of interest, but to also add headers and to group variables.
- ✦ The primary function of the Column statement is to provide a list of variables for Report to operate against, and these variables are listed in the order (left to right) that they are to appear on the report.
- ✦ In addition to listing the variables, you can do a number of other things on the Column statement as well. For instance you can use a comma to attach a statistic to a variable. The default statistic is the SUM.
- ✦ Parentheses can be used to create collections of variables or statistics.

To create a Detailed Report

Proc Report Data= YLP. Labs nowindows headline headskip;

Column Lbtest Lbnrind;

Run;

- The option Headline adds a line after the column headings and the Headskip option adds the blank line.
- The way to control which variables are outputted, is to use the COLUMN statement. This statement is similar to the VAR statement in Proc Print. It determines which variables are going to be in the report and in what order the variables are displayed.
- While choosing the variables we need to pick at least one character variable to create detailed report , if we pick all numeric variables then by default summary report would be created,

Proc Report Data=YLP. Labs headline headskip nowindows;

Column Patid Lbtest;

Run;

- Default Spacing between fields = 2 blanks
- Default Justification (=Alignment): RIGHT for Numeric Fields, LEFT for Character Fields
- If no format specified, then Proc REPORT uses Best9. for Numeric Fields, $w. for Character Fields (w=width).
- Default Width= Format width. It is quite easy to upgrade the spacing width by adding a width specification to the define statements

Proc Report Data=YLP. Labs Headline Headskip Nowd;

Column Subjid Site Age;

Define Subjid /Display;

Define Site / Display Width=4 Right;

Define Age / Display 'AGE' Width=3;

Run;

- 'AGE' column title was added to the DEFINE statement. This title overrides the label in the descriptor part of the input data set.

To create summary report:

Proc Report Data=YLP.Dmads nowindows;

Column Patid Race Ageyr;

Run;

- Rather than listing the values in the input data set, it sums the values. This is because the two variables (Patid and Ageyr) are numeric.
- When all the variables in the input file are numeric, Proc Report does SUM as a default, to avoid having the sum of numeric variables, one or more of the input variables must be defined as DISPLAY.

Using the Define Statement

- The Define statement lists the name of the column to which it applies and the attributes (following a '/') that are to be used. A primary attribute of the DEFINE statement is the 'type' of column. The type refers to how Report is to handle the variable.
- Each variable has a default type. However it is usually a good idea to include a Define statement for each column even if all of its desired attributes are the defaults.
- In a DEFINE statement, you specify the variable name followed by a slash and any options for that particular variable.

Syntax of Define Statement: *Define Var_Name / Usage_options Options 'style_attributes';*

In Define statement, the word after the slash specifies the define type for that column. The valid define types are Display, Order, Group, Analysis, Across, and Compute.

- ***Across:*** Creates a column for each unique value of the variable.
- ***Group:*** Creates a row for each unique value of the variable.
- ***Analysis:*** Calculates statistics for the variable. This is the default usage for numeric variables, and the default statistic is sum.

- ***Display:*** It creates one row for each observation in the data set. This is the default usage for Character variables.
- ***Order:*** Creates one row for each observation with rows arranged according to the values of the order variable.
- ***Computed:*** Define the item as a computed variable.

The DISPLAY option forces each observation to print. Furthermore, it is good programming practice to always define each variable that is in the output report. The following is an example of how to use the DEFINE statement.

Proc Report Data=YLP.Dmads (Keep=Patid Ageyr) NOWD;

Define Patid /Display;

Define Ageyr /Display;

Run;

Customize the appearance of a report item:

1. ***Format=*** Assign a SAS or user-defined format to the item.
2. ***Order=*** Order the values of a group, according to the specified order.

- ***Data:*** Orders values according to their order in the input data set.
- ***Formatted:*** Orders values by their formatted (external) values (Default).
- ***Freq:*** Orders values by ascending frequency count.
- ***Internal:*** Orders values by their unformatted values, which yield the same order that Proc Sort would yield.

3. ***Spacing=*** Define the number of blank characters to leave between the column being defined and the column immediately to its left.
4. ***Style=*** specifies the style element to use for column headings and for text inside cells for this report item.

A number of supplemental options can be used with the define statement to augment the display of the information. Some of these other options include:

- ***Format*** applies the standard SAS formats to the column,
- ***Width*** sets the column width,
- ***Noprint*** suppresses printing that column.

- ***Flow*** Text that is wider than the 'width=' option wraps within the block
- ***Statistic:*** Statistic to be calculated (analysis variables).
- ***Descending:*** Reverse the order in which PROC REPORT displays rows or values of a group, order, or across variable
- ***ID:*** Specify that the item that you are defining is an ID Variable, ID ensures that you can identify each row of the report when the report contains more columns than will fit on one page.
- You can replace the label as the ***column heading*** by specifying the new heading in quotes. The slash (i.e. '/') is the line break symbol used to force the heading to wrap lines.

Using Define type GROUP:

Group is used for the consolidation of rows, usually for summary purposes.

```
Proc Report Data=YLP. Labs headskip nowindows Split='|';
Column Patid Visid Lbproc Lbtest;
Define Lbproc / Group 'Lab|Procedure';
Run;
```

Split is to control the line breaks in the column headings

Using ACROSS with group

You can transpose rows into columns by using the ACROSS define type. In this example LBPROC is defined as an across variable. As a result a column will be formed for each distinct value taken on by LBPROC.

```
Proc Report Data=YLP. Labs headskip nowindows ;
Column Patid Visid Lbproc Lbtest ;
Define Lbproc / Across ;
Run;
```

Task: Execute each piece of code; observe the changes in the report.

Data vitals;

Input Subjid Visit Vsseq Vstest$ @@;

Datalines;

101 1 0 SBP 101 2 1 SBP 101 4 3 SBP

101 1 0 DBP 101 2 1 DBP 101 3 2 DBP 101 4 3 DBP

101 1 0 HR 101 2 1 HR 101 3 2 HR

;

Run;

Proc Report Data=vitals nowd; *Column Vstest Visit;* *Define Visit / Order* **Order=data**; *Run;*	*Proc Report Data=vitals nowd;* *Column Vstest Visit;* *Define Visit / Order* **Order=Internal**; *Run;*
Proc Report Data=vitals nowd; *Column Vstest Visit;* *Define Visit / Order* **Order=Freq**; *Run;*	*Proc Format;* *Value Visfmt 0= 'Screening'* *1= ' Randomization' 2= ' Dosing'* *3= ' Follow Up';* *Run;*
Data Vitalf; *Set Vitals;* *Format Visit Visfmt.;* *Run;*	*Proc Report Data=Vitalf nowd;* *Column Vstest Visit;* *Define Visit / Order* **Order=Formatted**; *Run;*
Proc Report Data=Vitals nowd; *Column Vstest Visit;* *Define Vstest /Order* **Order=internal;** *Define visit /Order* **Order=data**; *Run;*	*Proc Report Data=Vitals nowd;* *Column Vstest Visit;* *Define Vstest /Order* **Order=data**; *Define Visit /Order* **Order=internal**; *Run;*

Using the Break /Rbreak Statements

- Two statements allow you to insert breaks into a report.
- The BREAK statement adds a break for each unique value of the variable you specify, while the RBREAK statement does the same for the entire report.

Syntax of Break, Rbreak statement:

BREAK Location Variable / Options;

RBREAK Location / Options;

Location has two possible values: 1. Before 2. After

Options:

- Summarize -- To calculate sum
- Skip -- To leave a blank line between unique responses
- OL -- Draw a over line on the statistics
- UL -- Draw an underline below the statistics
- Page -- Present each unique value on a different page
- DUL -- Draw Double Under Line
- DOL -- Draw Double Over Line

Applying Breaks

```
Proc Report Data=YLP. Labs headline headskip nowindows;
Column Lbtest Lbrn Lbnrlo Lbnrhi;
Define Lbtest / Group 'Lab Test';
Define Lbrn / Display;
Break after Lbtest / Summarize Skip OL UL;
Rbreak after / Summarize Page DUL DOL;
Run;
```

Using Compute Block

Compute Block allows the use of most DATA step statements, logic, and functions, and through the use of the compute block you can modify existing columns, create new columns, write text, and many more.

The compute block starts with the COMPUTE statement and terminates with the ENDCOMP statement. Usually the compute block is placed in the REPORT step after the DEFINE statements.

The syntax of the compute block:

compute <location> <report_item> </ options>;

one or more SAS language elements

endcomp;

Using the LINE Statement

One of the more interesting programming statements within the compute block is the LINE statement. This statement is roughly analogous to the PUT statement in the DATA step and can be used to introduce lines of text into the report.

a blank line has been inserted AFTER each level of the grouping variable (LbProc)

compute after Lbproc;

line '---';

endcomp;

Adding Lines of Text

The LINE statement can also be used to add lines of text either at the top or bottom of the report. The LINE statement is more commonly used to add lines of text at specific locations in the report.

In the following example the text is written as a footnote at the end of the report. We can specify the options BEFORE and AFTER to indicate the location, and since in this case no grouping variable appears on the COMPUTE statement, the AFTER applies to the whole REPORT.

Computing Columns Based on Statistics.

It is often necessary for body mass index (BMI) to be included in Demography listings. Body Mass Index is calculated as weight (kg) divided by height squared (m2). The COMPUTE statement can be used to derive this variable and then display it in the final listing.

```
Define BMI / left computed format=6.2 "BMI*(kg/m^2)";
compute bmi;
BMI = weight / (height*height);
endcomp;
```

Creating Flag variables according to abnormal results

The COMPUTE statement can be used in PROC REPORT to attach flags to abnormal values. These types of output are commonly produced for listing ECG, Vital signs and Lab results. The SAS code below attaches High/Low flags to heart rate values outside the range.

It is important to ensure that the DISPLAY option is included on the variables used in COMPUTE blocks. In this example, the heartccd (Heart rate clinical concern code with value 'H' for high and 'L' for low) and heart (Heart rate in beats per minute) variables are used in the COMPUTE block. It is also necessary to list these variables prior to the computed variable in the columns statement. Finally, the "character" option will need to be used on the COMPUTE statement as heartpci is a computed character variable

```
Define heartccd / display noprint;
Define heart / display noprint;
Define heartpci / left computed width=8 "Heart*Rate (bpm)";
Break after subject /skip;
Compute heartpci / character length=20;
        if heartccd in ("H" "L") then heartpci=trim(left(heart))
|| " " ||trim(left(heartccd));
        else heartpci=trim(left(heart));
endcomp;
compute after _page_ / left;
        text1="H=High, L=Low";
        line text1 $108.0;
endcomp;
```

Varying Footnotes by Page

For tables that span multiple pages, a common practice is to put a standard message such as "See last page for footnotes" at the bottom of each page except the last, and a complete listing of all footnotes at the bottom of the table on the final page. This can help to conserve page space if there are numerous footnotes. The code below shows the use of the COMPUTE and LINE statement to add footnotes in this way.

The significant lines in the code are the “after” and “after _page_” options in the COMPUTE statement. The “after” option executes at the end of the table; the “after _page_” executes at the end of each page of the table.

```
compute after;
        hold = "x";
endcomp;
compute after _page_ / left;
        length text1 text2 text3 text4 $ 108;
        If hold="x" then do;
        text1="Message1"; text2=" Message2"; text3="
        Message3";      text4=" Message4";
end;
        else text1="See last page for footnotes.";
        line text1 $f108.; line text2 $f108.; line text3 $f108.; line
text4 $f108.;
endcomp;
```

Defining statistics creating the report as per mock shell:

```
Proc report data=YLP.Labs headline headskip nowindows split='*'
spacing=1;
column lbProc lbrn,(n mean) lbtest n (lbnrlo lbnrhi),mean ;
define lbtest / order 'Lab Test';
define lbrn/ display 'Lab Result' style=column [just=left
cellwidth=25%];
define lbnrlo/ display 'Lab test * Result Normal Low' style=column
[just=center cellwidth=40%];
break after lbtest/ summarize skip ol ul;
rbreak after/ summarize dul dol;
Run;
```

Nothing in life is to be feared.
It is only to be understood.

Marie Curie

STEP 17

SAS/GRAPH

In clinical trials we need to Present Data in (Graphs/Figures), Graphical Way, for this we use two Procedures:

1. Proc Gchart   2. Proc Gplot.

These two Procedures belongs to SAS/Graph Product

1. Proc Gchart -- Charts like Hbar, Vbar, Pie, Star, Donut Etc.,
2. Proc Gplot --

- ✦ Scatter plot
- ✦ Line plot
- ✦ Odds-Ratio plot
- ✦ Box-plot
- ✦ Kaplan-Meier plot (KM Plot)

Proc Gchart (GCHART Procedure)

PROC GCHART supports RUN-group Processing, which means the Procedure executes the group of statements following the PROC statement when a RUN statement is encountered additional statements followed by another RUN statement can be submitted without resubmitting the PROC statement the Procedure stays active until a PROC, DATA, or QUIT statement is encountered.

The GCHART Procedure produces vertical and horizontal bar charts, block charts, pie charts, and star charts, donut charts, Vbar3d, Hbar3d, Pie3d charts.

You can use bar charts to graphically display the distribution of a variable's values, average value of a variable for different categories, total value of a variable for different categories etc, When using the

GCHART Procedure, specify the physical form of the chart, identify a chart variable that determines the number of bars to create (Categorical) and identify an analysis variable to use for calculating statistics that determine the height (or length) of the bar.

By default, the height, length, or size represents a frequency count (N).

General form of the PROC GCHART statement:

Proc Gchart Data= YLP. Dmads;

Vbar Race;

Run;

Quit;

If the chart variable is character, bar or slice is created for each unique variable value. For numeric chart variables, the variables are assumed to be continuous unless otherwise specified. Intervals are automatically calculated and identified by midpoints. One bar or slice is constructed for each midpoint. To override the default behavior for numeric chart variables, use the DISCRETE option in the HBAR, VBAR, or PIE statement.

The DISCRETE option produces a bar or slice for each unique numeric variable value, the values are no longer treated as intervals.

Proc Gchart Data= YLP. Dmads;

Vbar Race/Discrete;

Run;

Quit;

By default, the statistic that determines the length or height of each bar or size of pie slice is a frequency count (N). To override the default frequency count, you can use the following HBAR, VBAR, or PIE statement options:

Proc Gchart Data= YLP. Dmads;

Vbar Race/ Discrete Sumvar=Ageyr;

Run;

Quit;

- ***SUMVAR=*** analysis-variable ***TYPE=***MEAN | SUM
- SUMVAR=Identifies the analysis variable to use for the sum or mean calculation
- TYPE=specifies that the height or length of the bar or size of the slice represents a mean or sum of the analysis-variable values.

To Present the Average age by Race

```
Proc Gchart Data= YLP. Dmads;
Vbar Race/ Discrete Sumvar=Ageyr Type=Mean;
Run;
Quit;
```

If we want to present Race wise Age in the 3D-bar chart and we want only Two Bars for Race1, 3.

```
Proc Gchart data=YLP. Dmads;
Vbar3d race/ Sumvar=Ageyr Midpoints=1, 3;
Run;
Quit;
```

While creating Pie or Pie3d Charts we can specify some more options like: Fill=, Explode= etc. You can use the ***FILL= option*** to specify whether to fill the pie slices in a solid (FILL=S) or crosshatched (FILL=X) pattern.

You can highlight individual slices of a pie chart by moving them away from the rest of the pie with the ***EXPLODE= option.***

```
Proc Gchart data=YLP. Dmads;
Pie Race / discrete sumvar=Ageyr type=Mean
        Fill=X Explode=2 Slice=Inside;
Run;
Quit;
```

```
Proc Gchart Data=YLP. Dmads;
Pie Race / Discrete Sumvar=Ageyr Type=Mean
          Fill=S Explode=2 Slice=Arrow Coutline=Green;
Run;
Quit;
```

GPLOT Procedure

You can use the GPLOT Procedure to plot one variable against another within a set of coordinate axes.

General form of a PROC GPLOT step:

```
PROC GPLOT DATA=SAS-data-set;
PLOT vertical-variable*horizontal-variable </options>;
RUN;
QUIT;
```

While creating Charts/Plots, we use the following statements to create the Figure/Graph as per mock shell:

- Goptions (Graphical Options) Statement
- Axis statement
- Legend Statement
- Symbol
- Pattern
- Title Statement
- Footnote Statement

GOPTIONS Statement: specifies graphics options that control the appearance of graphics elements by specifying characteristics such as default colors, fill patterns, fonts, or text height.

Graphics options can also temporarily change device settings.

General form of the GOPTIONS statement:

GOPTIONS graphics-options;

To reveal the devices provided by SAS:

Proc GDevice;

Run;

To use the specific device as per standards or client specification we can use DEV= Option. The ***DEVICE=*** (or DEV=) graphics option in the GOPTIONS statement specifies the graphics device

Goptions Dev=JPEG (We generally use PNG, CGMOF97L, JPEG, GIF)

AXIS statement: modifies the appearance, position, and range of values of axes in charts and plots. The AXIS statement controls the location, values and appearance of the axes in plots and charts.

Different options we use in Axis statement:

A. Axis scale options:- **Order=** (*value-list)*

B. Appearance options: **COLOR=***Axis-color*

LENGTH=*axis-length <units >*

OFFSET= (*n1,n2)*

WIDTH= *thickness-factor*

C. Tick mark options: **Major= , Minor=**

D. Text options: **LABEL= (angle= height=)**

SPLIT="split-char"

VALUE= (text-argument(s))

Legend Statement: Modifies Appearance, Position of legends generated by Procedures that produce Charts and Plots.

A. ***Appearance Options***

- ***ACROSS=*** Number-of-columns
- ***CBORDER=***Frame-color
- ***FRAME***

B. ***Position Options***

POSITION = (<BOTTOM | MIDDLE | TOP>
<LEFT | CENTER | RIGHT>
<INSIDE | OUTSIDE>)

C. ***Text Options***

- ***LABEL=*** *(*text-argument(s))
- ***ORDER=*** (value-list)
- ***VALUE=*** (text-argument(s))

SYMBOL statement: Specifies the shape and color of plot symbols as well the interpolation method for plot data. You can use the SYMBOL statement to define plotting symbols draw lines through the data points, specify the color of the plotting symbols and lines.

General form of the SYMBOL statement:

SYMBOL n options;

The value of n can range from 1 to 99. If n is omitted, Default is 1.

SYMBOL statements are:

Global -- Once defined, they remain in effect until changed or until the end of the SAS session. Additive -- Specifying the value of one option does not affect the values of other options.

You can specify the plotting symbol you want with the VALUE= option in the SYMBOL statement:

VALUE=symbol | V=symbol

Selected symbol values are Plus (Default), Diamond, Star, Triangle, Square etc

You can use I= option in the SYMBOL statement to draw lines between the data points. (I=interpolation)

Selected interpolation values:

- ***JOIN*** ---Joins the points with straight lines.
- ***SPLINE*** -- Joins the points with a smooth line.
- ***NEEDLE*** -- Draws vertical lines from the points to the horizontal axes.

Symbol value=dot Interpol=needle;

Modifying the SYMBOL Statement:

Set the attributes for SYMBOL1. S***ymbol1 C***=blue ***V***=diamond;

You can cancel a SYMBOL statement by submitting a null SYMBOL statement.

To cancel all SYMBOL statements:

Goptions reset=symbol;

PATTERN Statement: Controls the Color and Fill of patterns that are assigned to areas in charts and plots.

TITLE Statement: Adds Titles to graphics output

FOOTNOTE Statement: Adds Footnotes to graphics output.

Adding Titles and Footnotes: You can use TITLE and FOOTNOTE statement options to modify the characteristics of text strings.

- ***COLOR=***color | C=color
- ***FONT=*** type-font | F=type-font
- ***HEIGHT=*** n | H=n

Many of life's failures are people who did not
realize how close they were to success
when they gave up.

Thomas A. Edison

STEP 18

DOCUMENTATION & STANDARD OPERATING PROCEDURES

Different documents we use while performing SAS Clinical Programming.

Biostatistics and SAS Clinical Programming team needs to maintain these documents for tracking programming, project status, as well as to ensure timely delivery of the project.

1. Study Personnel Sheet

This Excel sheet gives a clear picture about all the people involved in this project, this document should contain the following information.

- Name
- Signature
- Initials
- Start Date
- End Date
- Study Role (Developer, Validator, Lead Programmer Etc)

II. Project Specific Training Record

We need to make sure that all the personnel working on a project should be capable of working on that specific data. To ensure this we provide them Project specific training and the details are recorded in Project specific training record.

- Participant Name
- Job Title
- Employee Code

- Signature
- Date of Training
- Method of Training (Live, Remote).

III. Project Delivery Plan

While starting on a Project, it is a good practice to prepare a sheet with all the required ADS and TLF names and understand their complexity, which is going to develop and validate, how much time one requires to develop and validate a Report, when we can deliver the Reports etc.,

Project Delivery Plan should contain the following details:

- ADS/TLF Number
- ADS/ TLF Name
- Module (Safety, Efficacy)
- Complexity (Simple, Medium, High)
- Status of Creation (Yes, No)
- Developer Name
- Development Status (Completed, Ongoing)
- Validator (QC) Name
- QC Status (Completed, Ongoing)
- Estimated Hours
- Development actual hours
- Validation Actual Hours
- Planned Delivery Date
- Delivery Date
- Delivery Status (Delivered/Not Delivered)
- Delivery/Issue confirmation Date
- Comments Received Date
- Resend Date
- Sign off Date
- Final Status

ISSUE LOG

While working on the project we may get several issues or a doubt which needs to be clarified within our team or sometimes with the client. If we have an issue needs to be addressed by client we will raise that issue in ISSUE LOG. This Issue log is like a bridge between us and the people working on the same project at client side like statisticians and data managers. Issue Log should contain the following information:

- Name of the ADS/TLF
- Finding
- Resolution
- Comment
- Status (Closed/Open)
- Issue Raised By
- Date Raised
- Assigned To
- Date Resolved
- Issue Resolved By

Weekly status Report

To track our performance and to update the client on our work status we should send him weekly status report. This will ensure that we are progressing on the project as per our committed time lines. This document should contain following information:

- Report Created By
- Reporting Period (From date – To date)
- Activities Planned/ Activities Executed
- Points For Discussion
- Inputs Required from Client
- Risk Status/ Risk Warning
- Identified Earlier (Yes/No)
- Expected Impact on the Project

VI. Defect Tracker

All the mistakes committed by developer or Validator needs to be tracked and maintained in a separate document in order to guide the Clinical SAS programmers.

- Date of Development/QC
- Developer ID/Name
- Validator ID/Name
- Defects (Internal/External)
- Defects Stage (QC Log, Consistency Review)
- Defects By (Developer/ Validator)
- Module (Safety/Efficacy)
- Activity (ADS,TLF)
- ADS/TLF Name
- Defect Category
- Defect Type
- Units (How many defects found)
- Defects Criticality (Critical/Non Critical)
- Accuracy Percent

Defects are classified as:

A) Programming Errors

B) Cosmetic Errors

Defect Type	Example of Defect	Critical/Non critical
A1.Algorithm related issue	A1.Incorrect logic for calculation of last observation carried forward (LOCF) leading to incorrect results	Critical
A2. Non-conformance to Statistical Analysis Plan (SAP)	A2. All subjects from test drug data set included in the analysis instead of 'Intent to Treat'/subjects with dosing records	Critical
A3. Non-conformance to programming Specifications	A3.Programming is not done as per the Specification	Critical
A4. Non-conformance to QC and Validation Procedures	A4.Process not followed (E.g. Not using Proc Compare to QC the derived datasets.)	Critical
A5. Non-conformance to analysis dataset specifications	A5 Variable format is different from the spec documents (E.g. Date format is not programmed as per the spec document)	Critical
A6. Occurrence of Warnings/Notes in the log file	A6.Warnings in log file such as 'Merge statement has more than one dataset with repeats of BY value'	Critical(depends on the type of warning)
A7. Incorrect Variable declaration	A7. Assigning a numeric value to character variable and vice versa	Critical
A8. Incorrect assumption of variables/ formulae	A8.Incorrect interpretation of the specification given in the SAP	Critical

B1.Coding standards not followed	B1. Keywords (PROC MEAN etc.) should be written in capital letters etc.	Non Critical
B2. Incorrect Titles, Footnotes, Page numbers and Page Setup	B2.Title for Demographic table is T1.2, however, it was captured as T1.6	Critical
B3.Spelling Errors	B3.Spelling errors seen in clinical terms, headers, footers, titles etc.	Non Critical
B4.Truncation of text and variables	B4.Truncated or incomplete titles, headers, footers, notes etc.	Non Critical(depends on the reporting variables)
B5. Non-conformance with List of tables(LOT)/Table of contents(TOC)	B5. Incorrect TLF names , TLF numbers etc.	Non Critical

VII. Tables transition sheet

To track ADS creation, Table, Listing, and Graphs creation we maintain a spread sheet which will gives us updated information about the status of the particular ADS, TLF.

- TLF Number
- TLF Name
- ADS Used
- Status
- Remarks
- Update
- Tables transitioned for programming
- Transitioned Tables Accepted by Team Lead
- Assumption Made on Tables.

VIII. Minutes of Meeting

To update the project status and to resolve or discuss the issues, it is common practice t have meeting with client twice weekly. After the discussion it is a good practice to document the discussion in a word document share it among the team. This document is called minutes of meeting. Minutes of meeting should contain the following information.

- Date of meeting
- Subject
- Attendees : from Clinitrial
- Attendees : from Client
- Discussion Points
- Minutes Circulated By
- Action Item
- Responsibility
- Target Closure Date
- Actual Closure Date
- Status (Open/Closed)

IX. Programming and QC Record

In this spread sheet we maintain the details of programmer who is responsible for development and for validation activities, If there are any modifications in the ADS, TLF programs we maintain version control and modification history.

- ADS/TLF Name
- Developer Name
- Version Number
- Developer Signature
- Development Date
- Validator Name
- Signature
- Version Number
- Date

X. Project Status Sheet

Project status spread sheet will give you the update on the project status at a glance.

- Table Number
- Table Name
- Unique Table /Repeat Table
- Creators Initials
- Creation Status
- QC Status
- Validator Initials

Standard Operating Procedures

While working on SAS clinical Programming we are supposed to follow specific Standard Operating Procedures to make sure those programs written in our organization meets our organization standards as well as regulatory standards.

STANDARD OPERATING PROCEDURES:

- SAS Programming Guidelines
- SAS Program Development
- Analysis Dataset, TLF Creation
- Validation and QC guidelines
- Statistical Analysis Plan
- Determination of Sample Size, Power
- Generation of Randomization Schedule
- Decoding Treatment Code
- Standard Directory Structure

SOP Contents:

- Objectives
- Scope
- Responsibilities
- Abbreviations
- Procedure
- References
- Annexure

For example, Let us take SAS Program Development SOP:

1. Objectives:

To describe the procedure for creating SAS programs following certain mandatory guidelines. This procedure is to ensure that all activities within Biostatistics for the Design and Development of a SAS program are in compliance with all applicable regulations, guidelines and Standard Operating Procedures (SOPs).

In particular it also ensures that Statistical Principles for Clinical Trials E9 and Good Clinical Practices E6 of the ICH guidelines are adhered to.

2. Scope:

This SOP applies to programs written to access, create and update data throughout the data life cycle (e.g. procedures which calculate values, load data, etc.) in Biostatistics in our organization.

3. Responsibilities:

The Senior Programmer /Project leader is responsible for ensuring that all programmers comply with this SOP.

4. Abbreviations:

BS	:	Biostatistics
CO	:	Clinical Operations
QA	:	Quality Assurance
DM	:	Clinical Data Management
ADS	:	Analysis Data Set
TLF	:	Table Listing Figure

5. Procedure:

6. References

6.1 ICH GCP guidelines

7. Annexure

SAS Programming Guidelines

I. General Programming Approach: Certain overall programming approaches have historically led to higher quality and productivity. All SAS programs that are developed within the Biostatistics and Programming department should in accordance with this SOP.

1.1. Standard Header Box: All SAS programs developed for Analysis and Reporting of Clinical Study Data and Quality Control of Associated Outputs, require an accurately completed standard header box.

This header must appear prior to the first line of SAS code and will contain the following information:

- Client's name and study protocol number.
- Project code.
- Program name.
- Program location: The location need only detail the directory path from after the project level onwards (e.g. PROGRAMS\TABLES).

- Program purpose: This should provide enough detail to inform a reviewer as to the overall purpose of the program, and should contain references to any relevant information from the SAP, protocol, e-mails or any other documents contained within the study files.
- Operating system and SAS version used.
- List of output files and permanent datasets created, including location. The location of the output files or permanent datasets need only detail the directory path from after the project level onwards (e.g. PROGRAMS\TABLES). If a non-standard directory structure is being used, then the full directory path must be presented.
- Name of Programmer, who created the program.
- Modification history.

1.2 Standard Directory Structures: This gives us an idea where our documents and output need to be stored. Some organizations maintain a separate SOP for Standard Directory Structures for Filing and Documentation.

1.3. Portability of Programs: Code should be as portable as possible in order to simplify internal system changes and to help ensure functionality on client systems. All programs should be as simple, straightforward and short as possible. Language features that are experimental should be avoided.

1.4. Single Programs to Create Multiple Outputs: To ensure consistency, a single program that makes good use of macro processing and/or dataset manipulations should be used to create closely related outputs. For example, a group of adverse event tables that are subset by different background characteristics should be produced within the same SAS program if possible.

1.5. Project Initialization Program: A single project initialization program should be used to establish Libnames, Global options, Global macro variable assignments, common titles and footnotes, etc. Chaining of format libraries and macro libraries should be specified in this file, and the chaining should first search the work directory. Chaining refers to the ability to search multiple locations in a particular order, and facilitates using program-level, project-level, protocol-level, client-level formats and macros.

1.6. Formats: Standard formats required for creation of analysis datasets, tables, figures and listings should be created centrally, i.e. in FORMATS.SAS, rather than within individual analysis dataset, table, figure or listing programs.

Format catalogs created by Data Management should be copied to a Biostatistics and Programming directory and a separate formats catalog should be created and maintained to store additional Biostatistics and Programming formats.

1.7 Commented Out Code: Our SOP states that commented out code should be removed prior to formal QC. Such code must be deleted, rather than left in a disabled state, to reduce noise and uncertainty within the program. This does not apply to the documentation of SAS code or the definition of macro variables.

1.8 Version Control: There is a regulatory requirement to version control all computer program code and related documentation. A program version number does not increment until changes are required after the associated output has been sent to the client (i.e., after each deliverable).

All programs must contain a standard header box and the header box must be up-to-date with the current version of the program.

II. PROGRAM READABILITY

2.1. Use of English: SAS programs should be always written in English to allow easy exchange of work across all locations

2.2. Lines and Spaces: Multiple statements should not appear on a single physical line (i.e., one statement ending in a semi-colon on each line). At least one blank line should be left between each section of code, procedure or data step. Where possible, all code should be visible within the width of the program editor window.

2.3. Indentation: It is recommended that sufficient indentation is used within the SAS code. The number of spaces by which to indent is left to you, but it should be enough to assist the readability of the SAS code. Indentation must be used for any subordinate processing (e.g., DO Loops, SELECT statements, %MACRO statements, etc..). An END, OTHERWISE or %MEND statement should always line up to match the corresponding DO or %MACRO statement.

2.4. Documentation of Code: Programs should be modularized into logical blocks of code, with each block being appropriately commented. Sufficient comments should be included to allow someone other than the original programmer to understand, run and update the program code. It is important that comments should always add value to the program, and they should not just state the obvious.

2.5. Dataset, Variable and Format Conventions: Each dataset must have a sensible name and must be explicitly specified on each data step and PROC statement.

2.6. Sub-setting Datasets: Temporary datasets should be as concise as possible and should only contain the variables and observations necessary for the program to execute without error. This can be achieved by using WHERE, KEEP and DROP statements when accessing datasets. It is far more efficient to use WHERE, KEEP and DROP statements when inputting a dataset rather than outputting a dataset - this avoids unnecessary processing of unwanted variables

2.7. Macros: Macro keyword parameters should always be used rather than positional parameters. This eliminates the chance of getting the macro invocation incorrect, as keyword parameters can be used in any order. Unless necessary, the use of GLOBAL variables should be avoided within macro code, if GLOBAL variables are used, sufficient documentation should be included within the code to clearly explain their use.

2.8. Filenames and SAS Options:

If filename statements are required or SAS options need to be changed, they should be assigned at the top of a program. There are some occasions when SAS options will need to be changed during the code execution (e.g., producing graphical output, outputs generated within a macro), but this should be kept to a minimum.

III. ELIMINATING ERRORS

3.1. Hard codes: Patient specific programming code, or programming code which alters the values of data, for any reason, thereby making them different from the values in the original source database are hard codes. This does not include programming code used to create derived variables or process data handling conventions , However, it does include programming code that assigns specific values to an individual patient's derived data (e.g., IF PATID = 904 THEN AGE=57).

Hardcoding would require us to deviate from SOP Writing of Computer Programs for Analysis and Reporting of Clinical Study Data and Quality Control of Associated Outputs, and must be avoided.

In certain extreme circumstances a hardcode may be necessary and, in those cases, a SOP deviation form must be completed and signed by the client. A comment must clearly identify the hardcode and must include the word "HARDCODE" on all relevant program lines, to allow for an automated search for all hard coding.

Example: Date of birth obtained after database lock hardcoded below:

If Patid= 904 then Birthdt = "18jan1957"d; *HARDCODE;

3.2. SAS Options: Options that constrain error detection or reporting should generally not be used. Included are NOFMTERR, NOMERROR, and NOSERROR. Sufficient documentation must exist within the code if any of the options that constrain error detection are used. The logs from final program runs should be of a manageable size, and thus should not use SYMBOLGEN, MACROGEN and MLOGIC options. These options, however, may be useful during individual program development and testing. MPRINT and SOURCE2 options should be used, especially when using macros or redirecting LOG output to an external file.

3.3. Standard User Generated LOG Messages:

Standard messages should be written to the LOG file using PUT statements for any conditions not controlled by the program logic.

Examples: *Put "ER" "ROR: Patient missing key information" Pt=;*

Put "WAR" "NING: patient missing drug start date" Pt=;

3.4. Character/Numeric Conversions: It is generally not acceptable to have messages in the LOG referring to the conversion of character variables into numeric and vice versa. This can be avoided with the use of INPUT and PUT functions.

3.5. Logical Operators: Brackets should be used for clarity and accuracy when using multiple logical operators (e.g., AND, OR and NOT) within a SAS statement. Without the use of brackets, mixtures of logical operators may function in different ways depending on the order in which they appear within the code. Note that an AND statement is resolved before an OR statement when code is processed internally within the SAS system.

3.6. Merging Datasets: A BY statement should always follow the MERGE statement. MERGE statements without an accompanying BY statement will, in most cases, lead to incorrect merging. A common source of error when using the MERGE statement occurs when the same variables (other than the merge by variables) appear on more than one dataset. In this case, the variable from the last dataset in the MERGE statement will overwrite the variable(s) from the other dataset(s). Clearly, careful use of DROP, KEEP and RENAME statements can prevent obtaining incorrect data in merged datasets.

Another incorrect use of the MERGE statement is trying to perform a many to many merge (i.e., if more than one dataset has multiple occurrences of a BY variable, SAS will not merge the two datasets correctly). This type of merge does not result in an ERROR or WARNING statement being added to the LOG file, although the NOTE statement below will be added: NOTE: MERGE statement has more than one dataset with repeats of BY values. The LOG file should always be checked for any MERGE statement notes and/or errors.

3.7. Mutually Exclusive Conditions: Ensure that complete logic is being used, i.e., that all possibilities for a data item are included within the statements. Examples of this are including a final ELSE in complex IF-THEN-ELSE code or using an OTHERWISE statement in a SELECT - END construct.

3.8. Missing Values: In addition to a period/full-stop, missing values can be represented by a combination of a full period and a single alphabetic character (e.g., .z). In order to avoid ignoring missing values by accident, it is best to write code that allows for all possible representations of a missing value.

3.9. Dataset Maintenance: The name of each temporary dataset containing data manipulations should be unique throughout the SAS code. This will assist in the development of the program, as it will enable the programmer to review each temporary dataset separately. This will also ensure that a program that runs with errors will not produce any output or results, as temporary datasets will not be created after the point within the program that the error occurs. If the same dataset name was being used throughout a program, the previous dataset created prior to the error occurring would continue to be used.

Validation and QC guidelines

INTRODUCTION:

This guideline provides details on how to perform validation of SAS programs, how to QC the output from such programs and how to QC other deliverables such as ADS, TLFs.

DEFINITIONS:

The term 'programmer' is used throughout to denote the person responsible for producing the original derived dataset or statistical output (Developer, Main Programmer), while 'QCer' is used to refer to the person performing the QC (Validation Programmer). The programmer and the QCer could be either a statistician or a Biostatistical programmer.

PROGRAM VALIDATION:

All programs produced during the reporting process should be written in accordance with Programming Guidelines. This applies to all programs written to determine or QC protocol violators and study populations, and all programs written to create or QC derived datasets, tables, listings, figures or any other statistical output. Before providing outputs to the QCer for review, the programmer should ensure that the program log is free of errors and all significant log messages are justifiable. The programmer should also check that the layout of the output is consistent with client specifications, no spelling errors exist in the output, the correct analysis population has been used and the numbers in the table make sense. This list of validation checks is not exhaustive, and it is suggested that the programmer refers to the standard list of QC checks to be applied to their output before submitting it for QC.

ALL OUTPUTS:

- Layout, titles and footnotes are consistent with client specifications
- Correct analysis population has been used
- Spelling correct (titles, footnotes, column headers, format etc.)
- Correct units of measure are used
- Consistent use of capitalization in titles and footnotes
- Consistent use of full-stops in footnotes
- Correct data formats have been used

- Number of decimal places is correct
- Change data (e.g. change from baseline) is calculated correctly (i.e. in the right direction)

TABLES ONLY:

- Summary statistics presented to appropriate number of decimal places
- Alignment is correct (e.g. summary statistics aligned by the decimal point)
- Appropriate wrapping over pages (e.g. summary statistics for a particular variable are not split over two pages)
- Total rows and/or columns are used when needed and are correct Percentages total correctly and correct denominator is used Cumulative tables accumulate correctly
- Population Ns are correct for all treatments at all visits
- Missing data and categories with no events are presented correctly.

FIGURES ONLY:

- Sensible LINE and SYMBOL options have been chosen (i.e. it is possible to differentiate between treatment groups).
- Axes have been labeled correctly, have units where appropriate and have a sensible scale
- Time points specified on axes agree with those presented in any matching tables.

WHEN DO WE QC?

It is recommended that QC is initially performed prior to sending the first draft version of the outputs to the client, unless the client has specifically requested to see a un-QC'ed version.

Messages to be checked in the log window:

- ERROR
- WARNING
- Lost Card
- SAS went to new line
- Numeric to Character conversion

- Character to Numeric conversion
- Variable Uninitialized
- Dataset with zero observations
- MERGE statement has more than one data set with repeats of BY variables
- W.D format was too small for the number to be printed
- Statement is not valid or it is used out of proper order
- Unbalanced quotation marks
- Referenced variable not found in the dataset
- length has already been defined
- Invalid argument to function
- Unknown
- Truncated

Proc Compare

Proc Compare is a SAS procedure which provides the programmer with a simple facility for comparing two datasets. While the procedure is capable of providing exhaustive listings of the differences between two datasets, it is frequently the case that the programmer is simply interested in confirming that two datasets are the same.

For example, a programmer may compare an output dataset to a previous version of the same dataset to verify that changes to the code which produced the dataset have had no unintended consequences. When accuracy of results is critical, datasets are often "Double programmed". The specified output is independently constructed by two separate programmers and the results are then compared.

Proc Compare generates the following information:

- Whether matching variables have different values.
- Whether one data set has more observations than the other.
- What variables the two data sets have in common.
- How many variables are in on data set but not in the other?
- Whether matching variables have different formats, labels or types.
- A comparison of the values of matching observations.

Proc Compare Syntax

Proc Compare <Base= Compare= Option(s)>;

BY <Descending> variable-1 ..;

ID < Descending> variable-1 ..;

VAR variable(s);

WITH variable(s);

Run;

Proc Compare Selected Options

- Brief – suppresses the four default summary reports (data set summary, variables summary, observation summary, and values summary) and produces a short comparison summary.
- Listobs – lists all observations found in only one data set.
- Listvar – lists all variables found in only one data set.
- Maxprint=Total | (Per-variable, Total) – specifies the maximum number of differences to print (default is 50,500).
- Noprint – suppresses all printed output
- Nosummary – Suppresses the four default summary reports.
- Novalues – Suppresses the value comparison results report.
- Outbase | Outcomp | Outdif – Writes base | comp | dif results to output data set specified in the Out= option.
- Outnoequal – Suppresses writing observation to the output data set when all values in the observation are judged equal.
- Transpose – Prints the value differences report by observation instead of by variable.

Proc Compare Data=Old_data Comp=New_data Listall;

Run;

If we want t compare different Variable names, we use couple statements in proc compare those are ***Var*** and ***With*** Statements.

Proc Compare Data=Old_data Comp=New_data;

Var ***Subjid*** *Event;*

With ***Subid*** *Event;*

Run;

The comparison will only be done on the variables in the VAR statement. You may also have a reason that you only want to compare a few variables so the VAR statement is useful to restrict the comparisons to the ones you want.

The programmer often scans the Proc Compare output for a note at the bottom saying ***"No unequal values were found. All values compared are exactly equal."*** This is a mistake which programmer might not consider the data discrepancies.

Let us have a look at some of the common data discrepancies that occur in Proc Compare:

- Missing Variables
- Missing Observations
- Conflicting Types
- Mismatched ID Variables

In order to avoid these, it is a good habit the SAS programmer should develop. i.e., ***"know your data".*** Know what variables you have in each dataset and their types, Know how many observations are in each dataset and where they came from. Examine your datasets carefully to make sure they contain what you are expecting.

COMPARING VALUES

By default, we see just the first 50 differences. If we have a large number of variables with lots of differences, we may also get this message: ***NOTE: The MAXPRINT= (50,500) printing limit has been reached. No more values will be printed.*** You can override this with the ***Maxprint= option***.

For example, the following code would restrict the differences to 20 per variable and 1000 overall.

```
Proc Compare Data=Old_data Comp=New_data Listall Maxprint=(20,1000);
Run;
```

Dealing with the Values very Close but not EXACT

Sometimes we may look at output and wonder why there is a difference. For example, both datasets have a value of 5. However, when we look more closely at the data you see the first dataset really has a value of 5.000000001 and the second dataset is exactly 5. This is common when you have a derived variable where the two programs used a different combination of functions to do the calculations. It might also occur if the datasets were generated under difference operating systems as precision can vary.

Once you have confirmed these values really should be treated as equal, you just need to specify the ***CRITERION= option*** with a large number of decimal places.

Proc Compare Data=Old_data Comp=New_data Listall ***Criterion=.00000001****;*

Var Vsrn;

Run;

Your output will now show that the values were treated as equal but not EXACTLY equal.

ID STATEMENT

Adding an ID statement can provide additional information that may speed up the process to determine why you have differences.

Proc Compare Data=Old_data Comp=New_data Listall;

Var Vsrn;

Id Subjid;

Run;

BY STATEMENT

If you add a BY statement, you get the same proc compare results split out by each BY group. You can also add NOTSORTED to your BY statement if the data isn't sorted. A one-to-one match will be performed. You can also use the DESCENDING option if variables in the BY statement are sorted that way. Just specify DESCENDING as part of the BY statement immediately before the appropriate variable.

Check Your Understanding:

Answer the following questions to check your understanding (Technical and Clinical Domain).

- What are the Variables you derived in ADSL?
- What are the statements you used in ODS?
- What are the advantages of SDTM?
- Explain Difference between Proc SQL (joining) and merge Statement?
- What are all the efficacy and safety Tables you have prepared?
- What are all the reports you have created?
- What are all the statistical procedures you worked on to get p-value?
- Explain ODS Trace ON statement?
- What are all therapeutic areas you worked on?
- How do you validate your program?
- Have you ever seen a message in log window saying that more than one dataset has repeat of by variables?
- What are all the variables present ADAE dataset?
- Explain Difference between treatment emergent adverse events and treatment related adverse events?
- What are the documents you refer before writing a program?
- What is SAP?
- Explain about the Analysis population in your study?
- Explain LOCF? Describe a situation where you use LOCF?
- What is the purpose of Put statement?
- Why do you use Data _Null_?
- What is the purpose of Put function?
- What are the Options you use in Proc Report?
- How do you perform match merge?
- How many ways are there to create Macro variables?
- How many titles you can use in a report?

- What is Null Title Statement?
- What is the purpose of Trim function?
- Do you use Scan function? What is the length of the variable created by scan function?
- How do you create a Macro Variable in Data step?
- Why do you use Proc Printto?
- How do you Store Formats?
- Explain Xport Transport format?
- Explain Dim function?
- What is PDV? Explain?
- What are Automatic Variables, Explain with examples?
- What is the purpose of Nodupkey Option?
- Why do you use Noprint option?
- Explain Into Clause?
- Explain Symbolgen Option?
- What are the Notes checked in Log window?
- Explain Msglevel= option?
- Explain In= Variable?
- Explain First. Variable and Last. Variable?
- Explain Retain Statement?
- How do you perform Many to many merge?
- Explain _Error_, _N_?
- Explain Null hypothesis and its considerations?
- Tell me the situations where did you use Arrays?
- Explain Invalue Statement?
- Which procedures you use to create graphs?
- Explain the situation where you prefer proc SQL to Data step?
- Why can't we use datastep for many to many merge?
- Explain Translate, Tranwrd functions with example?
- Explain Flow option in Proc Report?
- Explain distinct clause, Count Clauses in SQL?

- How many ways u can remove duplicates?
- Differences between WHERE & IF Statements?
- Explain about Debugging?
- What is the difference between a FUNCTION and a PROC?
- Explain Fmtsearch?
- What has been your most common programming mistake?
- Do you observe any coding standards? What are they?
- Do you follow SOP? Explain SAS programming guidelines?
- Are you using the Macros provided by client or creating your own?
- Under what circumstances would you code a SELECT construct instead of IF statements?
- How do you debug and test your SAS programs?
- Explain Lag function?
- Explain Dif function?
- Explain Legend statement?
- Explain Axis statement?
- Combining datasets with multiple set statements
- Combining datasets with set statement but with common observations
- %Let is used in open code and within a macro, which value would be in effect?
- Data _null_ Vs Proc Report, which one you used?
- Explain the purpose of Mprint and Mlogic
- How do you Store Macros?
- Explain Functions used in Macros?
- Explain the usage of Sysfunc function?
- What is current project, therapeutic area?
- What is the primary objective and secondary objective of your project?
- What are all the data sets you dealt with?
- Give me some examples of derived variables you created?

- How do you create ADS?
- How do you validate your Program, Output, and Log window?
- How do you validate report created by your colleague?
- Have you worked on Efficacy tables? Name them?
- What is ITT population?
- What are the variables you derived in ADAE?
- What is Safety population?
- Explain the difference between Listing and Table report
- What is TEAE? How do you derive TEAE Flag? Explain?
- Explain Derived variables in ADVS?
- What is the primary variable in your study?
- What do you know about Serious Adverse Events?
- What is the primary end point and secondary end point in your study?
- Do you use Proc Ttest? Explain the situation?
- Do you use Proc Lifetest? Explain the situation?
- Explain a situation where you use Data step with Arrays rather than Proc Transpose?
- What is Baseline definition in your study
- What are all the problems you faced while validating tables and reports?
- What are the rows present in protocol Violation table?
- What is shift table? Explain?
- What are all the therapeutic areas you are exposed to?
- What is Correlation and Regression? Explain?
- What do you know about ADaM?
- What is Imputation? How will you impute data? Explain a situation?
- Explain Data structure of ADLB, ADAE, ADSL, ADVS, ADCM
- Explain Analysis of Co-variance?
- Explain the derivation of change from Baseline?

- Explain the program check list you follow?
- What is consistency review? Explain?
- How do you derive Visseqid (Visit Sequence Id)?
- How do you derive Lbnrind (Lab Normal Indicator)?
- Explain the process of creating Specifications for ADS?
- Explain the Validation methods you are implementing in the current project?
- How do you compare datasets? How do you compare variables in a single dataset?
- How much time will you take to create a Table, Listing, Graph, and ADS?
- How do you derive Visfwdid (Visit Forward Id)?
- What are the problems you faced during the project?
- How many raw datasets you have in your project? Name them?
- What are the graphs you generated till now? Explain the purpose?
- What are the considerations you check when picking a SAS/STAT procedure?
- Have you worked on SDTM mapping? Explain?
- What is censoring? When did you use censoring?
- Have you worked on survival analysis?
- How will you create Kaplan-Meier plot? Which variable is taken on y-axis and x-axis?
- There are 5 adverse events for a subject and has taken 1 conmed to cure one particular adverse event. How can you decide that conmed related to that particular adverse event?
- Explain Safety table cross checking?
- There are 10 deaths in Disposition dataset? How will you cross validate this 10 subjects in report?
- During development process, how will you ensure that your program is creating correct output?
- How would you perform the validation for the listing, which has 400 pages?

- Explain your role in CRT?
- Have you created Xport transport files? Explain the purpose?
- What is the definition of TEAE? How will you consider the whether the event is Treatment Emergent or not?
- Explain the layout of the AE table with an example?
- Explain difference between treatment emergent adverse events and treatment related adverse events?
- What is Issue Log? Explain some issues you faced while working on project?
- What are the challenges you faced when you first implemented CDISC standards?
- How do you validate SDTM domains created by you?
- Explain Catt, Catx functions?
- Difference between Local and Global macro variables?
- What do you know about 21CRF PART 11? Explain its Importance?

INDEX

D

E

F

N

O

Q

R

S

W

X

Y

www.ingramcontent.com/pod-product-compliance
Lightning Source LLC
LaVergne TN
LVHW090317160826
845684LV00001B/8

9798894759494